Deaf Esprit:

Inspiration, Humor and Wisdom from the Deaf Community

D1293452

Damara Goff Paris
And
Mark Drolsbaugh

Deaf Esprit:

Inspiration, Humor and Wisdom
from the Deaf Community

Published by: AGO Gifts and Publications
P.O. Box 17664
Salem, Oregon 97305

ISBN: 0-9673998-0-7

Library of Congress Catalogue Number: 99-65347

Acknowledgments

We would like to thank the writers who submitted their stories to AGO Gifts and Publications. We could not have achieved our vision without their wonderful stories.

Thanks also to the people who encouraged us—our friends, colleagues, co-workers, former college instructors, and the staff of DeafNation Newspaper.

Special thanks to Sharon Kay Wood and Trina Miller. Your wisdom, feedback and encouragement will never be forgotten.

And, of course, we must thank our spouses, Melanie Drolsbaugh and Joseph Paris, for the support they gave, and the time they sacrificed, toward the success of *Deaf Esprit*.

Table of Contents

People Who Inspire Us

About the Editors

About the Illustrator

Foreword

Deafness is probably one of the most interesting paradoxes we'll ever see in this lifetime. Is it a disability? Is it a blessing or a curse? Is it something to be proud of? It's impossible to define!

As you read this book, you probably won't find any easy answers to the questions set forth above, but you'll understand that each person must define their own experience relating to deafness.

In my years of editing and producing the national newspaper, *DeafNation*, I've seen many stories and columns designed to capture the essence of being Deaf. Over time, I've realized that deafness is something that has to touch one's life in order to be fully understood. One must experience, understand, and embrace a world that is marked with stunning visuals, sometimes violent clashes with the world around it, a sense of quiet desperation, and the marked desire to evolve into something more.

As described by the various contributors to *Deaf Esprit*, we've seen some marvelous progress being made in the Deaf world, and yet, we also see serious setbacks. At times, this may make one wonder, "Is it really worth it to be a Deaf person?"

It has been said that being deaf is an inconvenience, no matter what kind of positive spin you put on it.

Maybe that is true. Many of us continue to face discrimination in the workplace, as well as difficulty with access when using relay services. We continue to curse at our TTYs that are missing their keys, and stay awake all night just because the baby cry signaler broke down, and the replacement part will not be available for two more weeks.

We are shortchanged educationally because the system is inconsistent at best, and damaging at worst. We face serious deficits in how our communication needs are accommodated in the educational setting. Not to mention the invasive medical and technological advances in the areas of vaccination and cochlear implants. The medical eradication of deafness is probably only 10 years away. Don't get me started about having to order food at the local Taco Bell with paper and pen, and finding that the order is completely wrong because the cashier is functionally illiterate!

The continued obstacles that Deaf people face are enough to make a hard-core, left-hand-to-the-ear-with-right-fist-raised-Deaf-Power advocate walk away in disgust.

By now, you may be wondering, "What are you trying to tell me? Give up advocating for Deaf equality?"

Nah.

Life is inconvenient, period. Technological advances can't change that! The heart and soul of Deaf people cannot be eradicated by cochlear implants or other technology. Deafness isn't limited to the scratches on an audiogram, and many of us who have ever befriended a hearing person who thinks like a Deaf person know this.

Life is made up of unique, personal, and individual challenges, and if we tried to compare our frustrations to others, we'd be hard pressed to find one other life experience that we'd willingly trade ours for.

It's up to each of us to make positive opportunities in this life, regardless of whether we are Deaf, a cultural or ethnic minority, or disabled.

As evidenced by the writers of *Deaf Esprit*, many community members have decided to take their chances and make their opportunities, regardless of what the outside world tells them that they should or should not be.

Being Deaf can mean being whatever you want it to be. Life can be like a sweet smelling, beautiful rose to be shown off to everyone in the world.

As the stories in *Deaf Esprit* exemplify, people who are proud of their deafness are likely to feel that they have unlimited possibilities in life.

The incredible diversity evident in the contributors' views on deafness and it's impact on their lives makes reading this book a pleasure. I have learned, through my years of being an editor for a national newspaper, that shared stories and a variety of perspectives allows us to see the world it should be seen, a delightfully dizzying array of people, cultures, values, and expectations.

The editors of this book, Damara Paris and Mark Drolsbaugh, are very skilled journalists and writers. In the past, both have contributed regularly to DeafNation newspaper. Together, they have produced a book that encompasses a unique painting of a Deaf world that continues to defy any single or simple definition.

So, instead of trying to define deafness in any traditional or limiting way, I invite you to open the next page and experience it one exciting personal drama at a time!

May your journey into the paradoxical Deaf world be filled with fascinating twists and turns!

Marvin T. Miller
Editor-in-Chief
DeafNation Newspaper

Introduction

Everybody wants one thing: to be understood.
–Sam Scott

All of us, to one extent or another, want somebody to *understand*. To understand where we come from. To understand our diverse backgrounds and experiences, and how they have shaped us into the beings we are.

It is no different for those of us who are involved in the Deaf community. Most of us have gone through a plethora of experiences related to deafness. Some of us grew up Deaf. Some of us may have a parent, sibling, or friend who is Deaf. Some of us may work in the Deaf community. All of these experiences, in their own unique way, have a profound impact on us. And it is human nature for us to want to share these experiences, so that people will *understand*.

When Mark initially wrote and published *Deaf Again* in the summer of 1997, he was doing precisely the same thing; trying to get the world to understand deafness as seen through the eyes of someone who is Deaf. After a series of lectures and book signing events, Mark was pleasantly surprised to find that he wasn't alone. Everywhere he went, there was a considerable number of people who approached him with their own stories. Each and every person, he realized, has an incredibly powerful story to tell. The challenge, however, was finding a forum to present these stories to the world.

This is where Damara came in. Already one step ahead, she had developed AGO Gifts and Publications with the intent to publish original books, focusing on people from the Deaf community, including an impending biographical series of essays focusing on Deaf women in *Deaf Women in the Pacific Northwest.*

As fate would have it, Damara and Mark developed a professional relationship while writing articles and features for *DeafNation*, a popular, nationally distributed newspaper. They began corresponding on a regular basis and found that their goals and ambitions were surprisingly similar. Inevitably, they decided to team up and put together a book where many powerful Deaf stories would become available for everyone to enjoy.

Soon after, at the 1998 NAD Conference in San Antonio, Texas, the concept for *Deaf Esprit* became a reality. The book title, however, was a challenge. Many titles were tried and discarded, until finally one was found—*Deaf Esprit*. Esprit was derived from the expression "*esprit de corps*" which can be translated as "enthusiasm of the group for a specific cause" or "group community spirit." Hence, *Deaf Esprit* was named to encompass the contributors' enthusiasm for the Deaf community.

After the concept of *Deaf Esprit* was made public, stories began coming in from all over the United States. Damara and Mark got to work putting it all together, one submission at a time. Wendell Goff also joined the team to provide his artistic input for the book cover and the illustrations.

Finally, after months of editing, re-editing, computer crashes, tight schedules and red tape, it was done. *Deaf Esprit* has turned out to be an impressive collection of stories. They are touching, inspiring, and empowering. They show Deafness from a genuine, real-life perspective, as told by people who have been there. People who, like the rest of us, wish, and deserve to be, understood.

— *The Editors*

Deaf Identity

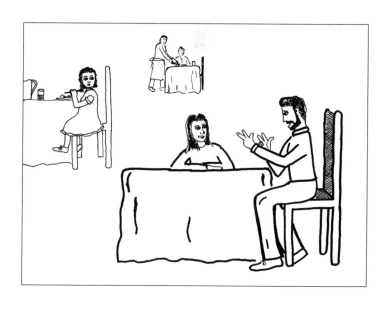

*Illustrated by Wendell E. Goff

I Am Five Years Old

By Rob I. Roth

I am five years old. I'm in a restaurant with my family. Bored and unable to follow the conversation, my eyes drift off to another table nearby, where four people are sitting. A man is moving his hands, gliding them gracefully through the air using an assortment of handshapes. He seems to be talking to his companions, but his mouth does not move like my father's. His mouth makes shapes that I've never seen before; they are very different from the mouth shapes my speech teacher uses. His face is animated. His eyes widen, then narrow. Sometimes his fingers come into contact with his eyes, then seemingly change shape in midair. He stops. A woman at the table begins to make similar movements with her hands. I stare. The man notices me, winks, and smiles. I smile back.

~~~~~~

I am seven. I'm on a school bus. The driver pulls away from the curb of Bell School, taking us all home. I've had a bad day. Earlier, I had been talking to my classmates, using my hands, when the speech teacher hit me on top of my hand with a ruler. When I began explaining to her, she hit me again, and then pointed to her mouth. I remember to put my hands behind my back and use my mouth to talk. It was a painful reminder. I forget about my sore hand on the bus as the kids draw me into their game of make believe; this time, I am a gangster with a machine gun.

~~~~~~

I am nine. I'm in class with Karen, Mary, Diane, Christopher and Bruce. We are paying attention to the teacher as she leads us through our lipreading lesson. Her mouth puckers to an "O" sound. Mrs. Welch shows us a picture of a ribbon: "BOW." Then she moves on to the next picture, a boat with oars: "ROW." And then... she does something that completely takes us by surprise. She goes to her desk, reaches inside for something, moves her hair behind her ear... and takes out her hearing aid. We watch in awe as she replaces a battery. We are dumbstruck. We look at each other and mouth: "Teacher–Deaf–same! Mrs. Welch–same–us!" It takes several minutes for her to calm us down. Later, at the bus ramp, we talk excitedly about Mrs. Welch. "We–grow–stay–Deaf!"

~~~~~~

I am eleven. It is near the end of the school year. My teacher, Mr. Teller*, informs me that next year I'll be placed in regular classes with hearing kids. I will not be with my friends in the portable classroom anymore. We will no longer be together and tell stories as we wait for the school bus, in our language of nasal voices, grunts and home signs. A few days later, I hit someone in frustration. Mr. Teller takes me aside and says, "If you don't behave, you go back with the dirty Deaf kids next year!" I become a model student until school is over. The following year, I rarely see my friends. A year later, I am transferred to my neighborhood school. I stop using my hands to talk.

~~~~~~

I am sixteen. I'm upset with my high school counselor, who has suggested I look into the National Technical Institute of the Deaf. He thinks it might be a good college for me. I tell him I want nothing to do with Deaf people.

~~~~~~

I am seventeen. I run into an old childhood friend, Ken, and we catch up on the news. He signs and uses his voice, and I find myself strangely comfortable with this. He introduces me to several old friends that I hadn't seen in years, as well as others that I had not met before. Some of them sign exclusively using their voice. I try to follow the conversation. Ken has to explain to me what each person is saying.

~~~~~~

I am nineteen, on spring vacation from college. I am driving to Washington, D.C., to visit Ken, who is attending the college for the Deaf, Gallaudet. I am nervous being around so many Deaf people. Will people like me? I know they sign, and I don't. I'm hard of hearing, and they are Deaf. While Ken is explaining to me what they are saying, I notice that those who don't use their voice have no patience with me.

~~~~~~

I am twenty-one. I am working as a teacher's aide in a summer school for Deaf children. The other workers are students from Gallaudet and NTID who are home for the summer. I hang out with them and enjoy their company, although I never fully understand their jokes (I always pretend to laugh at the right time). I begin to pick up signs, and a few friends are patient with me. When summer is over, I enroll in a sign language class at the YMCA. The teacher signs in English word order... I think this is easy. I secretly attend classes, telling only a few trusted friends.

~~~~~~

I am twenty-three. I am visiting NTID, thinking about going back to college for a Masters degree, and I knock on the door of a childhood friend who works there. He is in his office, along with someone else. Signing awkwardly, I fingerspell "h-i" to my old friend. He looks at the other person, shrugs, and signs "hearing-on-the-head." He is not aware that I know that sign. Discouraged, I keep my chin up, but leave shortly afterwards.

~~~~~~

I am twenty-five. I have moved to California, with plans to attend California State University at Northridge. They have a Deaf program there, and I have some vague ideas about designing educational materials for the deaf. I decide to take a sign language class at a community college, commuting from a friend's house until I find a place to live. The class book has a psychedelic cover, and is titled "Ameslan." Only one other person in the class is hard of hearing. We become friendly and decide to rent an apartment together. We discover that our new apartment complex has quite a few deaf people living there. We gather nightly at the hot tub. In our conversations, I find myself understanding signs more and more. We talk about our lives, our goals, what we will do tomorrow, and the upcoming Deaf Day at Disneyland. I grow comfortable with my new friends; comfortable talking with my hands.

~~~~~~

I am forty-eight. We are in a restaurant, my friends and I. We talk to each other in American Sign Language... laughing, teasing, serious, insulting, then laughing again. Our hands punctuate the air, while our faces underline the signs. Suddenly I notice a little girl, two tables away. She is sitting quietly at her table, staring at me. Her parents, brothers and sisters are all moving their mouths, talking. I wonder. I smile at her. She smiles back.

Rob I. Roth was born in Chicago, Illnois, and has recently moved from Seattle, Washington, to the San Francisco Bay area. He is currently the Chief Executive Officer of Deaf Counseling, Advocacy, and Referral Agency (DCARA). His stories "Boy Scout of America" and "Say the Word" were published in *Eyes of Desire: A Deaf Gay and Lesbian Reader.*

*Name changed to protect identity

"D" on the Nose

by Donna Platt

My sign name is "D" on the middle bridge of the nose. Naturally your first thought might be that I am referring to a certain part of the male anatomy. No, my name is not Dick. It is Donna, and I am not ashamed or embarrassed about my sign name. It is very special to me. I received this sign from Deaf children, who lived in Dumaguete, in the Philippines, where I served three and a half years as a Peace Corps Volunteer.

I grew up in a hearing school with no support service system or sign language. I had learned a few signs when I was 15, however, I began to learn on a daily basis when I entered into the NTID (National Technical Institute for the Deaf) at the Rochester Institute of Technology (RIT) in Rochester, New York, at the age of 18. While I was a student at NTID, my sign name was changed every year. Therefore, when I arrived in the Philippines and the Deaf children asked me for my sign name, and I decided to let them to go ahead and select one for me.

When the children showed me my new sign name, I was startled. I was going to ask them to think of another name, but then I thought, "Hey, I am in the Philippines now, and the American translation of that sign does not exist here. That sign looks good on them and it represents their culture."

I was tired of common sign names and I wanted my sign name to be original. In the Filipino culture, it is typical for both Deaf and hearing people to be fascinated with foreigners' noses because by Filipinos' standards, they were so big.

I used that sign name for five years while in the Philippines and during travels to Asian countries. I stopped using my sign name when I returned to the USA. After two and a half years in this country, I realized I missed my sign name. It was part of my identity. I noticed there were many unusual name signs in Seattle. I thought, "Why must I follow the established American Sign Language (ASL) standards for using my name sign?" Because I had been given so many common sign names, I wanted something different, something unusual that I could identity with.

After completing my graduate studies and moving to Seattle, I discussed re-using my sign name with a friend. Her response was that people would be flabbergasted, but that they would get used to it after a while. In Asian countries, my sign name was positioned at the tip of the nose. To minimize the confusion here in America, I changed my sign name a little by moving it to the middle bridge of the nose. At the time, I did not care what people thought, and I still don't.

My sign name has been the cause of some funny incidents. Here are some of my favorites:

I have a Peace Corps friend, whom I met in Nepal and who had learned Nepalese Sign Language as her first sign language. We unexpectedly met again at our graduate school orientation. I introduced her to a male friend of mine. Later, my friend came to me and asked me what was happening with my sign name. I realized that I hadn't warned her about the ASL translation of my sign name. She told me that earlier she had signed to a male friend, "Where D?" and he appeared to be shocked. She had exclaimed, "C'mon, you know where D!"

A week after the 1989 Deaf Way event, in the Gallaudet University Library, a Deaf man from Bangladesh was looking for me. He appeared to be agitated as he stood in the center of the room and signed, "Where D?" People were startled until the student employee, also from the Philippines, came to him and asked him to fingerspell out the word for "D."

My clients had a tour of the community center for the Deaf and Hard of Hearing led by a Deaf employee, Sally. * The clients realized that it was nearly time for their job search skills class to begin. They told Sally that they had to leave because "D would get mad." It was well known that I expected them to be on time for the class in order to prove their job readiness. Sally pointed to the restrooms, assuming that this is what the sign "D" stood for. The group said no, and that they had to leave at once because "D" would get mad. Sally became increasingly confused as she interpreted this to mean that the group needed to use the bathroom.

Although I left the Philippines thirteen years ago, I still have warm memories of my time there, and would not trade those experiences for anything. I am still happy with my sign name and have no regrets about it, because it gives me a unique identity. I don't intend to change it despite American sign name standards or what others may think. Of course, I still get puzzled looks from people when they first learn my sign name. Regardless, I give thanks to my friends and other people who have the courage to use my sign name.

Donna Platt currently lives in Seattle, Washington. She graduated with an BS in Social Work from Rochester Institute of Technology (RIT) and an MS in Educational Technology from Gallaudet University. She currently works part time in a variety of positions, including job developer, telecommunication access service trainer, and an instructor with the Washington State 9-1-1/TTY Education Program. She has written several articles for Peace Corps publications, and gave a presentation on double culture shock, which was published in the first Access Silent Asian national conference proceedings.

*Name changed to protect identity

Back to the Star

By Billy "Rusty" Wales

At the early age of one month, I became what many children and even some adults always dreamed of—a child movie star in Hollywood.

Six months later I was summoned back to the casting company for another movie. My mother innocently revealed that I was Deaf. "Deaf? Next, Please!" said one movie producer. Rejected, I experienced job discrimination as an innocent baby. His reaction was odd considering that there were no speaking lines in the movie.

Fast-forward a few years later to my elementary school, where none of the teachers could understand me. Nor could I understand them. They would not let me use my native language, the one I used to communicate with my older Deaf sister and our Deaf peers on the playground. Hearing kids in my neighborhood laughed and jeered at my funny voice.

I was literally at the height of my career, being paid more than I ever needed while I was still in diapers. After the rejection by the movie producer, my life plummeted to rock bottom in a world where no one could understand me.

I could have become a drunken "has-been" teenager like those child movie stars who grow up. What saved my life was American Sign Language—ASL. I am not kidding you! Here's my story:

St. Vincent Hospital, where I was born in 1944, happened to be located in Hollywood. The producer, who was seeking a baby to cast in his movie, "Three's a Family," came to visit the maternity ward at the hospital.

There were many newborn babies in the nursery, and I was among them. When one baby started crying in his cradle, other babies responded to the crying noises and started to cry as well. I was blessed with being congenitally Deaf, so I slept peacefully in that noisy room. The producer couldn't stand "crybabies" in his movie production, so he handpicked the baby with a happy face, not necessarily the pretty one. I happened to be that baby. Had the producer known that I was Deaf, he probably would have picked another one!

About eight years later, I attended a public elementary school. I sat in a classroom with other Deaf kids being taught by a hearing teacher who was long overdue for retirement. I sat through the class time clueless, never able to understand one single word our senior citizen teacher tried to teach. She expected too much from me in particular, because of my ability to talk orally and clearly. It was well known among the faculty that I was a product of an internationally famous clinic known for its preschool oral training for deaf children. My mother was a speech teacher at that clinic, so all of my teachers had unrealistically high expectations of me. If I failed to meet their expectations, for example, not being able to pronounce a "ch" word correctly, or not being able to read their seemingly deformed lips, then they called me a "brat" or an "underachiever."

One day, when I gave the verbal answer to my teacher's question in the class discussion, my teacher told me it was wrong. Then one of my classmates copied my answer and she correctly pronounced it. "Right!" said the teacher. I felt resentful as the girl with the ugly curly hair got the credit and smiled smugly at me. I did what any normal boy would do in that situation: I got mad.

"THAT'S MY ANSWER, YOU @#$&!," I said in sign language.

I ended up sitting on the dunce's seat in the corner. I also got my hands rapped with the teacher's ruler for using sign language, a taboo in the school with an oral philosophy.

After these incidents began to occur daily, I started to imagine that two different scenarios would play out after school. One scenario reflected what I imagined would happen to anyone else in my position, and the other scenario reflected what was actually happening at my home:

Scenario #1, a "Regular kid" coming home after school, Mom in the kitchen preparing dinner: "How was your day at school, honey?"

Regular Kid: "That girl copied my answer and gave it to the teacher in the classroom. She cheats all the time @#!& her!"

Mom: "Watch your language! You have to report this to your teacher."

Regular Kid: "I did! All she did was hit my hand with a ruler for using signs."

Mom: "What!? Did she touch you!? I have to report this to the principal."

Scenario #2 Rusty, a Deaf kid in a similar situation:

Mom: "How was your day at school, Honey?"

Me: "Fine!" (Avoiding talking more in my unnatural language)

Mom: "What's the matter with you— you look sad?"

Me: "Th-th-that kir-irl" (stuttering)

Mom: (correcting my speech) "g" not "k" "girl" (places my hand on her throat so that I can feel her voice).

Me: "j", oh ok "g"...j-irl, oh ok, "g-irl" (pronounced awkwardly).

Mom: "Correct! Now, what happened?'

Me: "Th-that j-irl copy me at s-s-skol–never mind!" (Walks away).

I had lost the momentum! It was too aggravating to try a hit or miss approach to make my point. Often I gave up during this constant struggle to communicate. I would rather be considered a fool than have to talk anymore with my Mom.

At that school, I was labeled as a troublemaker, or even mentally retarded, because I could not speak at the level of my Deaf sister. It was natural for her and very few other kids to learn speech. Perhaps, she loved to talk. Learning to talk was a matter of survival for her. I became a passive student. I saw no reason to participate when other schoolmates could parrot my answers. From child star to class dud! I sat in despair as life passed me by.

This concerned my parents. Although my sister did well in class, she had no social life or friends among the hearing pupils. Talking with them without using our native language was too difficult. My parents decided to send us to another school where Deaf children were allowed to converse in American Sign Language. It was a nerve-wracking decision for my parents. Not only because of the change to a school that employed a contrasting communication mode, but also because they would be sending their children to a residential school. Any loving parents would be hesitant to let their kids leave the nest prematurely. The most difficult part, for them, was that the philosophy of my mother's employer, was opposed to the philosophy of the residential school. My mother stood firm while all the faculty members around her gossiped, talking behind her back about how she was setting a bad example for other parents and consumers.

What happened for me, as a 12 year-old lad half-way through K-12, was a complete turnaround! I was finally allowed to express myself in my own way, in my natural communication mode, without hesitation about how to say a word right, and without stern corrections from a teacher. There were no more barriers to communication. My desire to learn was restored!

Sending my sister and I to a residential school did not alienate us from our parents. When we came home, we communicated even more with our parents, and as a result we became closer.

I came to adore some of the teachers at my new school. Some of them were Deaf. They were there for me everyday, and I wanted to follow in their footsteps. They provided me with options, and one of these was college. I went on to Gallaudet University and earned my Bachelor's, then to California State University, San Diego State University, and others for my advanced degrees. I have worked as a teacher, curriculum specialist, project director, assistant principal, rehabilitation counselor, telecommunications supervisor, and an administrator of a state agency. Along the way, with all of the highs and lows, I hope I have made some impact on other young Deaf children. I have come a long way from rock bottom by rebounding and leaping toward the star I once was in the beginning of my life. I thank the Lord for this divine invention called ASL!

Rusty Wales currently works as an administrator for the Utah Division of Services for the Deaf and Hard of Hearing. He received his MA from California State University, Northridge. He has published several stories in the *California School for the Deaf, Riverside, History Book* (to be released in the fall of 1999). Another story entitled "Can't You Sign? No Problemo!" will be published in a future edition of the *Chicken Soup for the Soul...with Disabilities.*

Anything Goes in Deaf Culture

By Mark Drolsbaugh

One of the best things about being a counselor is watching children grow and discover new worlds. It's even more fun when the kids find out that they have access to worlds they previously thought they'd never be a part of. It's like watching a slow, squirming caterpillar become an elegant, graceful butterfly that can fly anywhere it wants to.

Sharon*, age 12, recently transferred to a school for the Deaf. Although intelligent and attractive, she was painfully shy. She was well dressed, often wearing clothes that won the admiration of her peers. She was polite and respectful, but had trouble looking anyone in the eye. As it turned out, she had a significant amount of residual hearing; most people described her as "hard of hearing" instead of deaf. Her speech, although she didn't use it much, was rather clear. She signed slowly and haltingly, as ASL was obviously new to her. She had been placed in a hearing program earlier because people assumed her speech and hearing ability indicated she would thrive in the mainstream. Apparently, they were wrong. Constant failure and frustration had left her without any confidence in herself.

When Sharon first joined a peer discussion group, she barely participated. The other students' flying hands spewed ASL at a rate far too fast for her to comprehend. As co-leader of the support group, I did my best to get her involved in discussion, but after the initial "whazzup" and some icebreaker activities, Sharon would be left in the dust. It was going to be an uphill battle.

After about a month, however, Sharon began to make progress. Her constant exposure to ASL made a noticeable difference. Sharon had gradually picked up many signs and was able to sign for herself in class. Previously, teachers had to interpret what she was saying to the other students because she usually answered questions with a mix of voice and fingerspelling. Suddenly, she was beginning to sign on her own. She was finally making friends, as she met other students who were also somewhat hard of hearing. Not only did she find peers that she could identify with, but they also assisted her immensely in terms of language acquisition. They were able to code-switch between Sharon's world of lipreading and their world of ASL. They successfully built a bridge that Sharon could cross.

Armed with improved communication skills, Sharon was ready to participate in the peer discussion group. She wasted no time in bringing up a powerful issue.

"I feel bad that I'm deaf," she began, "Because being deaf means you can't sing or rap." She went on to describe her favorite rap stars, and lamented about how her hearing friends could become involved in music, while she was cut off from that world.

Despite having enough hearing to enjoy numerous rap stars, she was depressed because she couldn't follow in their footsteps. She would never be a famous performer.

"Have you ever seen Peter Cook?" I asked. Sharon said yes, as Cook had just wrapped up a two-week residency at the school. An internationally renowned Deaf poet and storyteller, Cook was poetry in motion, and a famous performer. Sharon's eyes widened as another student handed her a newspaper article that described Cook's ASL poetry and storytelling.

"He travels all over the world?" Sharon asked, incredulously. The other students nodded their affirmation. She shook her head in amazement, and then asked another question.

"But what about rap? I still can't rap, because I'm deaf."

"Have you ever seen CJ Jones?" I asked. Sharon said no, that she had transferred to our school after Jones had visited us. The other students quickly took the lead and told Sharon that Jones was an awesome Deaf comedian who includes rap in his repertoire. In a recent performance, he brought the house down with his brand of Deaf rap, entitled "I Can't Hear You, Say It Louder Now." In addition to his rap, Jones also raised the roof with his ASL rendition of the Stevie Wonder song "Part-Time Lover." Sharon's jaw dropped to the floor.

"Deaf people can rap?" she asked. "Really?"

"Of course!" said another student. Two other kids jumped into the conversation, disclosing how they were going to do an ASL rap at an upcoming talent show. They had rehearsed diligently and were ready to rock the house.

Wrapping up the discussion, I emphasized that the student performers' artistic endeavors didn't have to end there; if they wanted to, they could continue rapping in high school and college. The Gallaudet Dance Company and the Deaf performing group known as "The Wild Zappers" were cited as examples.

By this time, Sharon was smiling from ear to ear. The transformation was nearly complete. She had made the jump from a world of "I can't" to one of "I can." In the hearing world, she had always experienced the frustration of being one step behind her hearing friends, stuck in a world of "close, but not quite." In the Deaf world, she had learned that anything was possible.

This is not a knock on the hearing world. We all have to interact with it to one degree or the other, and we all do so in whatever way works best for us. However, the Deaf world is where many of us get that first taste of equality and success, and once you get that first real taste of accomplishment, you strive for more. Many people use that initial success in the Deaf world as a springboard for success anywhere. You've got to start somewhere, and there's no better place to do it than amongst your true peers. Sharon is just one of several students I've seen bounce back and take off once they've had that first taste, and I know there will be plenty more. Anything goes in Deaf Culture, and the sky's the limit.

Mark Drolsbaugh currently lives in Pennsylvania with his wife and newborn son. He wears many hats in the Deaf Community, including school counselor at the Pennsylvania School for the Deaf, an AIDS educator at the Community Center for Professional Services, and a newspaper columnist for DeafNation newspaper. He is the author of *Deaf Again*.

*Name changed to protect identity

The Closed Door

By Carrie Pierce

The door, it's closed
Resisting, it opens slightly
Just a crack
Its privacy reserved
Revealing just a sliver of light
Afraid of opening
Why, I'm not so sure

Behind the closed door
An unopened book
Sits, alone, in its corner
On the cover
Rests a purple heart
In it, a keyhole
Somewhere sits a key
The key that turns open
A story
That so desperately
Needs to unfold
Fragile pages remain unturned

Will the covers become layered with dust?
Or will time allow the fragile pages to be turned?

What Are You...Deaf?

By Carrie Pierce

As I look back on all my years growing up in the hearing world as a Deaf child, one of my worst memories is lip reading these exact words: "What are you.... Deaf?" When I sit down and analyze the situation, maybe those words were not so bad after all. In a way, they triggered the initial phase of my discovery that I am truly a Deaf person. While it took several years for me to develop this identity, that dreaded phrase was perhaps the most powerful catalyst to discovering it.

Growing up, as a child, I never told anyone about my deafness unless I felt it would cause more embarrassment by *not* telling people. I felt my parents made sure I was as "normal" as possible. Therefore, I always tried to pretend that I could hear so I could fit in. I always made sure that my hair covered my hearing aids. Because I was able to keep up by reading lips and I spoke only when someone asked me a question, people rarely noticed my speech problem. If they did, I wasn't aware of it.

As early as fifth grade, I had the dream of playing professional basketball in Europe. Men have the NBA here in the United States, but prior to the development of WNBA, women had to go to Europe to continue with basketball after college. Eager to get on the right path toward realizing this dream, I attended basketball camp for five years in a row at the University of Maine. Every summer I would pack up, never knowing whether my little secret would be discovered. Once I got on campus, I would be under the supervision of the coaches and players from the University of Maine women's team. These players also had the dream of making it to Europe—and three of them succeeded. They were my role models when I was a child. I admired them so much that I went to almost all of their home games, as well as a few that were out of state. The first year I attended camp was right after I completed fifth grade. It went well considering that I knew no one, except my second cousin who comforted me on those days when I felt homesick. My Deafness was not noticed at camp. I never told anyone, except for some of the friendlier coaches, as well as a few peers. I did well keeping up with everyone.

My second year was an entirely different story. Three of my closest friends from school had joined me. Keeping up with everyone was getting more difficult, particularly since I was a teenager and I was becoming more social. There were more places to go and more things to do. My peers talked non-stop about everything. As usual, one of my goals was to make it through the day without anyone finding out that I wasn't "normal." I hadn't told anyone I was Deaf. I just watched what everyone else did and followed along. I was able to keep up and understand just enough so that I looked like I knew what I was doing. But did I really know what I was doing?

One afternoon we gathered in the field house, which contained six basketball courts, side by side, encircled by an indoor track. We were doing the usual run of drills with Joe McGinley*, the assistant coach of the women's team (his brother just happened to be the head coach). I didn't like Joe from the start. His attitude really annoyed me and he didn't seem to care about anyone, or anything, except his job. Under normal circumstances, I would have called him Coach McGinley. But I didn't think he deserved that much respect.

During this particular drill, my roommate Natalie was in my group. Joe assigned us to do lay-ups, or at least that is what I thought he wanted. Nothing fancy, just lay-ups. There's nothing difficult about lay-ups—just four different steps, right? As usual, I copied what everyone else was doing. We continued doing lay-ups, but all of a sudden, everybody stopped. Joe started screaming and hollering. He was moving his lips so fast that the only word I could catch was "wrong." I knew the steps of a lay-up perfectly because I had reviewed the steps over and over again in my head. As he continued screaming, I thought I read the words, "run around the track." I assumed this meant that if we did whatever we were doing wrong again, we would have to run around the track. My turn came and went. I checked Joe's face, in hopes that I would see an expression that would mean that I had done it right. I looked up at him and he appeared to be very angry. I caught the word "run." So, I hit the track. When I finally got back to our court, he started yelling at me again. This time I read his lips perfectly. Never in my life had I been able to lip read a phrase so well.

"WHAT ARE YOU… DEAF? You were supposed to run around the court, not the track!"

My heart sank, my face went red, and tears began to fall. I could have melted into a puddle on that basketball court. He kept getting bigger and bigger, and I could feel myself shrinking. The phrase "What are you…Deaf?" echoed in my head. Am I Deaf? I thought it over quickly and gave him an answer.

"Yes, as a matter of fact I am."

He was so shocked that he didn't have anything more to say, and neither did I. But what could anyone say? I was relieved when someone blew a whistle and it was time for us to go to dinner. I don't think I could have taken the sight of his face a moment longer. Without hesitation, I ran for the door to meet my friends and told them what had happened.

My roommate Natalie, who had witnessed the incident, stayed behind to talk with Joe. Later on, she told me that she had made it clear to him that his behavior was inappropriate.

Somehow, I made it through the rest of the week without looking at Joe. I also managed to make the all-star team. But I couldn't have done it without my friends. They told all of my coaches that I was Deaf and I didn't have any more problems the rest of the week.

In the years to come, whenever my friends and I saw Joe at basketball games, we always gave him dirty looks. Often, a look of confusion would cross his face. I know that we looked a lot different than we did in sixth grade, but how could he not remember any of us?

For the next eight years, I continued to hide the fact that I was Deaf. I always knew that I wasn't accomplishing anything by hiding it. I just could never get myself to admit that I wasn't "normal." It wasn't until many years later that I realized that it is okay not to be normal because **there is no such thing as normal**! I slowly opened up and allowed people to become aware of my Deafness. A few years ago I learned to accept that I was Deaf. Now I am now able to tell people "Yes, I am Deaf," and feel pride when I say it.

Carrie Pierce is a Maryland resident. She graduated from Gallaudet with an MA in Family Centered Early Education. She worked as a Director at the local YMCA and has recently accepted a job in the field of education in Maine.

*Name changed to protect identity

The Impossible Ideal

By Jake McConnell

Recently, I wrote an article for a magazine that focused on the cochlear implant controversy. And sure enough, not long after the article came out, arguments popped up everywhere. In my own house. This is what happens when my hearing relatives get their hands on the stuff I've written. I am the family kook, and the family occasionally likes to check and see if my head is screwed on straight.

Basically, in the aforementioned article, I said that if an adult chooses to have a cochlear implant, that's his or her own business. No one should complain about it. When it comes to children, we could argue about this endlessly. Nonetheless, if a child already has an implant, it is imperative that the Deaf community accepts this child. Many children who do not succeed with the implant (I have stated many times that it does not make Joe Deaf become Joe Hearing) eventually drift over to the Deaf community. It is frustrating not to be able to fit in with the hearing world, and that would be compounded if a deaf child with an implant that failed found himself rejected by the Deaf community. My stance is pure and simple: if someone (adult or child) already has a cochlear implant, let it go. Welcome that person.

Although for the most part I have preached tolerance, I have precluded this concept with a disclaimer that my own personal opinion of the implant has always been, and still is, "no thanks." If you have or want a cochlear implant, that's fine with me. But I don't want one for myself.

This is where someone in my family took offense. Murphy's Law dictates that this relative is somehow going to read this article. For the sake of both our sanity, I'm going to give her a fictional name. Let's call her Jessica. Jessica definitely liked the article, particularly the way I showed acceptance for adults who have the cochlear implant. But she did not like the fact that I don't like it enough for myself. She also did not like my stance against implanting young children before they are old enough to decide for themselves. She immediately challenged me to validate my opinion.

I explained that it is in the Deaf world that I found professional success after years of frustration and failure in the hearing world. Unable to measure up to hearing ideals, I discovered the Deaf Community. ASL has opened up far more doors for me than hearing aids or speech therapy ever did.

Jessica, however, refused to acknowledge that Deaf Culture exists. And I objected and insisted that it did. The Deaf world has its own language, art, history and mores, I explained. I showed her some materials from National Association of the Deaf (NAD) and other Deaf organizations, and while she admitted that I had good points, they weren't good enough to influence her overall perspective.

Taking one last shot at it, I tried to explain to Jessica that Deaf Culture is as important to me as her religion is to her. How would she feel if mainstream society insisted she convert to the more dominant Christian religions? Jessica shook her head no and bristled, "That's different!" she said. Furthermore, she felt that every Deaf person, including myself, should jump at any opportunity to become more hearing. And the cochlear implant is a great way to start.

Quite frankly, I felt crushed. Jessica is a relative I love very much. When she thumbs her nose at Deaf Culture, she thumbs her nose at a very big part of me. I live, eat, drink, and breathe Deaf Culture. It is who I am. So it really stings when she rejects it.

Finally, Jessica said our whole argument was moot anyway. Unbeknownst to me, she had gone to a workshop on the cochlear implant and inquired as to whether or not I was a possible candidate for it. She was chagrined to find out that I was not a viable candidate.

I too felt chagrined. I was chagrined to learn that Jessica still feels a need to go out and fix me. I know that she does it out of love, and in her own way, she does what she thinks is best for me. Yet it still pains me that she does not see me as the successful person that I am. To her, I will always be the hearing impaired person in the family, the man who cannot hear. I am the man who needs to be repaired. The fact that I can survive and thrive in a world without sound is just too foreign a concept for her to accept. So she sets an ideal for me, an audist ideal which I cannot reach.

After all of the discussion that went on, I realized that there was no way I could have change Jessica's view any more than she could have changed mine. We called it even. We still love each other, and we joked to other relatives that we were "going for the throat" with this issue. Jessica plans to show my original article to other hearing relatives. And I think I'm going to lock myself in the basement before they come after me.

In retrospect, this was just an amicable argument between two individuals. But what do we, the Deaf Community, do to address this issue on a larger scale? It's not uncommon for many hearing people to look at things from an entirely audist perspective. The world of ASL and Deaf Culture is understandably incomprehensible to a lot of people. My argument with Jessica essentially ended in a draw and we agreed to disagree. But I would have lost entirely if I did not have NAD and a strong organized Deaf Community to fall back on. At one point in our argument, Jessica insisted I had no proof. When I told her about the recent NAD Conference, with it's many workshops and research findings presented there, Jessica was able to acknowledge a portion of it.

At this juncture, my only advice to the Deaf individual is to be more visible. In recent years, we've had a growing number of Deaf professionals. We need more. When the hearing world sees more Deaf CEO's, administrators, business managers, entrepreneurs, financial advisors and other professionals, they take notice. Our world is more likely to be recognized and respected if we are visible. There are still some hearing people out there who marvel at the fact that I can drive a car, let alone hold a steady job. So my plea is for Deaf people to keep striving for success in the world. Show them what you can do! Do everything possible to ensure that the next Deaf generation will build on and surpass your own successes. Then, and only then, when you insist there is a Deaf Culture will people listen. It's the only action I can think of.

One final thought—We are fortunate that there are many wonderful hearing people who do understand. Some of them advocate fiercely on behalf of Deaf Culture. They are a valuable resource. Often, they are the ones who can convince other hearing people (the ones who won't give me the time of the day) to give Deaf Culture a chance. I appreciate the help. You know who you are…and God Bless You.

Jake McConnell is a freelance writer from Long Beach Island, New Jersey. A self-proclaimed beach bum, he brings his trusty laptop to the edge of the surf and types away amidst a glorious sunrise. McConnell, who "prefers to keep a low profile," has had several articles published nationwide under a pen name.

Rock, Paper, Scissors

By Charlotte Wilhite

School children have been playing it for dozens, maybe hundreds of years. It's an interesting concept. Three separate entities, each stronger than one and weaker than the other. In the traditional game it goes like this: Rock beats Scissors, Scissors cuts Paper, and Paper covers Rock. In the math world, if A is greater than B and B is greater than C, then A must be greater than C. But it doesn't work that way in the game of Rock, Paper, Scissors. One has to think deeper, with more logic and creativity. Those are the rules, and kids love it.

Like thousands of children before him, our son, then 7 years old, was intrigued by the game. Because sign language is his mode of communication, the handshapes probably struck a resonating chord in his spirit. The excitement of chance, the equal possibility of beating or being beaten by other players, the satisfaction of bashing, chopping, or enclosing the hand of the opponent. It is thrilling! Nick had only been playing the game for about seven minutes when he started making up his own rules.

Nick preferred to have other handshapes appear unexpectedly. My Rock was easily overcome by his Ocean. Obviously it sank, he explained. My Scissors were torn up by his Tyrannosaurus Rex, which was hardly fazed by the small pecking motions the scissors made against the Rex's leathery skin. My Paper was burned up in his raging Fire. When I tried to play by his rules, he still won more often than not.

If the superiority of his handshape was not apparent, he would argue its merits. I tried to drown his Dragon in my Ocean, but he pointed out that Dragons could fly. Bears can climb Trees, but if Trees fall on them, they can run fast and avoid being hit. He was a master at the game, and had quite a boorish attitude about it, too.

One day he invited my sister Laura to play. Laura is quite competitive herself. Possessing a high level of intelligence and resourcefulness, she is a perfectionist who is used to winning. I warned my sister that Nick did not play by the traditional rules. Anything could pop up.

"But, Nick," she protested. "There are supposed to be only three choices." He was appalled.

"That's too boring!" said my son. "Other things can appear, too, like wind or animals," he explained. Laura thought a moment.

"You mean ANYTHING can happen?" she asked. Nick nodded enthusiastically. "O.K., then, we'll play it your way," agreed Aunt Laura.

In the first round, Laura produced a bent "two" handshape in her palm that she claimed could defeat Nick's Monster.

"That," she explained, "is a Bug, and it can eat ANYTHING."

"But bugs are little, tiny things," countered Nick.

"Not this one." Aunt Laura inched it toward the Monster, making bug-mouth motions. "It is a HUGE bug that can eat your Monster."

"Fine." Nick was amused and gracious. "You win that one."

Next round, Laura put a sideways "four" into her palm that she described as "a Machine that can destroy ANYTHING. Especially that mountain."

"This is a gigantic mountain."

"This Machine can ruin it." The "four" started moving forward.

"Okay, but it will take it a long time," Nick conceded, laughing.

Then Aunt Laura made two fingers stand up in her palm. "This is Superman, and he is stronger than ANYTHING."

"But my Rocket is very, very, FAST!"

"Your Rocket can not hurt Superman. He is faster than a speeding bullet."

Nick paused, then brightened. "I will beat you for sure next time!"

The following round, Nick signed "Green." Laura asked what that was all about.

"It's the Green Rock that makes Superman feel weak."

"Well, it can't do anything to my Hole," she said smoothly. "This Hole is so big that EVERYTHING falls into it." The Hole approached the Green Rock and sucked it in. Both of them, and me too, were laughing hysterically. When we regained our composure, Nick looked at Laura with respect. "You are a very skillful player!" He said.

"Yes," said Aunt Laura smugly. "You have met your equal!"

In future matches, I would try to incorporate Laura's creations into my own game. However, Nick's mind had been simmering with new handshapes, and he had defined them more clearly. My Machine was too slow to destroy his Cheetah, fastest animal on earth. His Earth wasn't affected by falling into the Hole, because the Earth was in space anyway. A disproportionate amount of times, it seemed to me, the Green Rock would somehow show up to weaken my Superman.

One time we were playing a rousing three-way game with Claire, Laura's 7 year-old daughter. The rhythmic nature of the game and the uncertainty of our opponents' options had overwrought us into frenzied laughter. Suddenly, Nick signed "God." Claire and I looked at each other, shocked.

"Well, nothing can beat God," we agreed. For the next few hands we each selected the Deity simultaneously. This was uproarious at the time but would become dull if we continued this way indefinitely. Finally we compromised on the acceptance of one guideline: you can only choose God one time in the game.

Unless, of course, someone comes up with a crazier and more interesting way to play...

Charlotte Wilhite is a registered nurse, a part-time interpreter and has had several photographs published in *Memory Maker's Magazine.* She lives with her husband Max and their nine-year-old son, Nick, in Ft. Worth, Texas. Nick lost his hearing after contracting meningitis at age 10 months.

Stories That Inspire A Smile

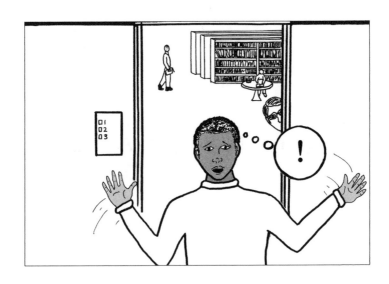

*Illustrated by Wendell E. Goff

The Library

By CJ Jones

We are thrilled to have the opportunity to include a story from CJ Jones, a world-famous Deaf comedian who has entertained Deaf and hearing audiences for years with his marvelous brand of comedy. CJ is also a writer, director, producer, teacher, and founder of the world's first Deaf television network, Sign World TV. In addition to starting up his own network, he has also served as Executive Director of Hands Across Communications, a non-profit organization which provides tutors to help mainstreamed students improve their academic and social skills. CJ's impressive career has included appearances on Sesame Street, A Different World, and a number of popular videos for Deaf and hearing children. He has traveled with the National Theater of the Deaf and performed in Children of a Lesser God on Broadway. Most recently, he co-starred in The Ride, a critically acclaimed short film. We are honored to be able to provide Deaf Esprit readers with an excerpt from CJ's comedy show, CJ Jones: The Living Cartoon. — The Editors

Know what? The other day, I decided to catch up on some deafness-related literature. Where else would I go but the Deaf Studies section of the local library? That is, if we had a Deaf Studies section. I wasn't too sure, so I approached the librarian at the desk.

"Do you have any books on Deaf Studies?" I asked.

"Yes," said the librarian. "Just take the elevator up to the third floor, it's the second aisle on the right."

Eager to get started, I got into the elevator and pressed "3". The elevator lurched forward awkwardly, and then slowly made its way up to the third floor. It came to a jarring stop, throwing me slightly off-balance. When was the last time they serviced this old relic, I wondered. 1947? Geez. I couldn't wait to get out of there. I made a mental note to take the stairs on the way down.

Suddenly—the horror! I was on the third floor and the elevator door would not open. Oh no! I knew I shouldn't have hopped into that rickety old bucket, it was probably powered by a wind-up rubberband. What was I gonna do?

Okay, the first step was to tell myself not to panic. So far, so good. The second step was to look for a way to get the heck out of there. Hmm. All right, I found my ticket out. It was an emergency phone. Yeah, right! An emergency phone with no TTY. Not too accessible for a Deaf guy. Now what? I began to press the "3" and "door open" buttons repeatedly. I was having no luck, the door still wasn't opening.

At this point, the third step was to panic. I started pounding on the door, screaming all the while.

"Help! Lemme outta here! I'm stuck! I'm too young to die! Get me outta this freaking tin can! Helllllllllp!"

After what seemed like an eternity, the elevator suddenly shook loose and slowly creaked its way back down to the first floor. This time, the door opened and I sighed in relief. I made a beeline to the librarian and gave her a piece of my mind.

"Hey," I motioned to her. "You need to get that elevator fixed. I was stuck up there on the third floor!" I wiped the sweat off my brow, still shaken from the experience.

"Did you look behind you?" The librarian asked. "On the third floor, the rear door opens."

My face flushed with embarrassment, and I wished I could shrink down to the size of an ant. I was ready to slip through a crack in the floor and find a rock to hide under. Glancing upwards towards the third floor balcony, I realized a whole bunch of people were sitting there. These people had been treated to an unexpected and loud performance.

From their vantage point, the elevator door had opened and they had seen the back of my head as I was screaming and pounding on the opposite door. They must have been wondering when the men in the white suits were going to come and take me away. Oh, man. I've had embarrassing moments before, but this one topped them all.

"Would you still like to check out our Deaf Studies section?" The librarian politely inquired.

"Uh, no," I said. I wasn't going back. I smiled awkwardly and inched my way out of the door. I would find the Deaf Studies section another time, in another library, in another state. And next time, I'd take the stairs.

Too Young

By David Kessler

I'm a hearing man who never knew any sign language before meeting my wife many years ago.

In my experiences with the Deaf community, I have found Deaf people to be quite a bit more open about certain topics that tend to embarrass hearing people. However, I was quite surprised one night while dining out with my wife and her friends. I followed the conversation as best I could. As the topic turned to husbands, I tried hard to hide my thoughts as one woman, with her 3-year-old son sitting beside her, casually told the group that she and her husband had not had sex in eight years. The "x" handshape coming down across the cheek meant, "sex." This was one of the few signs I was sure of.

Later, I asked my wife about the conversation, repeating the part about "Eight years without sex." She didn't see the problem.

"What about the boy?" I asked her.

"What do you mean?" she said. "He's much too young to shave."

David Kessler currently lives with his wife in California. He graduated from California State University, Northridge, with a Multiple Subject and Special Education Teaching Credentials from CSUN. Both he and his wife run a website called DeafMall.net (www.deafmall.net), where people can do their Deaf-related shopping.

Deaf is Smart

By Trina Miller

For several years, I worked with Deaf youth as a counselor, in a school setting. There was a girl that I worked with, on and off, from the ages of 11 through 14. Early on in our sessions, she frequently talked about becoming a hearing person when she got older. She would not accept any opposing discussion on this topic, so determined was she to become hearing. She often listened to the radio for "practice." Time went by, and she never did become a hearing person. She stopped talking about that dream. However, she could not stop dreaming about a world that she would fit into as a Deaf individual.

One day, years later, she came to our session looking upset. She poured out the story of how alone she felt in her hearing family, and how her family members had refused to learn sign to improve communication with her. Often, she felt left out of family activities and isolated emotionally from the people that she wanted to be close with. Over time, she had interpreted her family's behavior to mean that they did not consider Deaf people to be as smart as hearing people. She felt that it was obvious that Deaf people are more intelligent because they use sign language to communicate. In the typical, absolute fashion that I had come to expect from her, she resolved to move into the Deaf school permanently, and sever all ties with hearing people forever.

Seeking to challenge her perception that all hearing people think they are superior to Deaf, I carefully reminded her that I was hearing. She dismissed me summarily with, "You are smart, for a hearing person. You can sign."

Trina Miller has provided a variety of professional services to the Deaf community over the past ten years, including mental health counseling, and interpreting. She helped to develop the first relay service in Alaska, and has also written for several publications, including *Deaf Nation Newspaper*. Trina holds an MS in Rehabilitation Counseling from Western Oregon University, and is currently pursuing her doctorate in Deaf Education at Lamar University in Texas.

The Deaf Apprentice

By Billy "Rusty" Wales

There was once a Deaf apprentice named Joe Wails,

Whose rights to sign language were denied by the townsfolk.

No gestures were used by his master, who chewed on rusty nails,

To hapless Joey, "pellet" and "mallet", on the lips looked alike.

So one day his bearded blacksmith boss shouted a rapid-fire writ

As he held the red-hot horseshoe with the tongs over the hot fire pit:

> "I will take the shoe over to thar' anvil;
> When I nod my head, ye hit it!"

Joey, not knowing what to do with the hammer or which "it" was to hit,

Thought: "What did he say? Oh, he is repeating 'hit, hit, you #&@!'
Gosh, he is mad now; I think he says, 'head'"!

Joey just did what he was told with a full swing of his mighty fist.

Swooosh...smash! There fell the bearded master, now lifeless.

Lo and behold, that deaf lad now had become the village blacksmith!

Rusty Wales currently works as an administrator for the Utah Division of Services for the Deaf and Hard of Hearing. He received his MA from the California State University, Northridge. He has published several stories in the *California School for the Deaf, Riverside History Book* (to be released in the fall of 1999). Another story, entitled "Can't You Sign? No Problemo!", will be published in the future edition of the *Chicken Soup for the Soul...with Disabilities.*

Valentine's Day Surprise!

By Leonard A. Marshall

Ellen and Leonard (Lenny) Marshall, who are both Deaf, will always remember the Sunday morning of February 14, 1999. Ellen and Lenny exchanged gifts that day, which was unusual because they usually exchanged simple, but endearing greeting cards. But wait, we are getting ahead of the story! Let's go back a bit for a beautiful story of how two people touched each other's hearts in an amazingly inspirational way.

In early January, Ellen went to a jeweler to have an "ILY" tie tack made especially for Lenny. She explained to the jeweler in precise detail how she wanted the tie tack to be made, with a unique Deaf touch to it.

Ellen's order was ready by the end of January. Thrilled with how beautiful the tie tack was, she showed it to everyone in the neighborhood, except Lenny, of course. She was so excited that she couldn't wait for Valentine's Day to arrive. She was like a child eagerly waiting for Santa Claus on Christmas Eve.

While all of this was going on, Lenny spontaneously decided he wanted to get Ellen an "ILY" pendant for Valentine's Day. He made an "ILY" shape with his hand, traced it onto a piece of paper, and then scanned it on the computer. With his "ILY" design in hand, he went searching for a jeweler. The first place he went to turned out to be closed, because the shop had gone out of business. Fortunately, there happened to be another jewelry store not too far down the same block.

Lenny walked in the jewelry store and inquired about whether they could do custom-made jewelry. To his delight, they could. He pulled out the "ILY" design that he had created and asked if a pendant could be made according to his specifications. The jeweler nodded yes, breaking into a wide smile as the arrangements were taken care of. Unbeknownst to Lenny, it was the exact same jeweler Ellen had gone to for the "ILY" tie tack.

When Valentine's Day finally arrived, Ellen and Lenny were in the midst of a wonderful weekend vacation. They were staying at the famed West Baden Springs Hotel, touring and taking in the sights of Southern Indiana. Little did they know how much they were about to surprise each other on this special Valentine's Day morning!

Ellen and Lenny exchanged colorfully wrapped gifts, and Lenny opened his first. His jaw dropped. There it was—an "ILY" tie tack fashioned in a shockingly familiar design. Lenny was beside himself, and asked Ellen if she had gone to a certain jeweler. Ellen said yes, and immediately wanted to know how Lenny knew where she had gotten the gift. Amazed beyond words, Lenny motioned to her present, encouraging her to open it right away.

Now it was Ellen's turn to be surprised. Peeling off the red wrapping paper, her eyes lit up in surprise. It was an identically designed "ILY" pendant! The only real difference between the two gifts was the color of the stone, as Lenny's was blue and Ellen's was red. Each color specifically chosen to represent the recipient's birth month. It was amazing. Lenny and Ellen vowed that before retiring at night, they would touch the thumbs of their "ILY" jewelry together as a symbol of their love.

Driving along the side roads of West Baden later that day, Lenny and Ellen talked about the incredibly romantic coincidence of their identical gifts. Lenny laughed and wondered how the jeweler managed to keep a straight face the whole time. Perhaps he was Cupid in disguise. As Lenny and Ellen drove off into the sunset, they beamed with joy, incredibly in love with each other.

Leonard Marshall lives in Indianapolis, Indiana. He graduated from the California School for the Deaf and attended Gallaudet University. Active in the Deaf Community, Leonard is a retired printer who currently uses his free time as the Secretary of the Indiana Association of the Deaf.

The Parental View

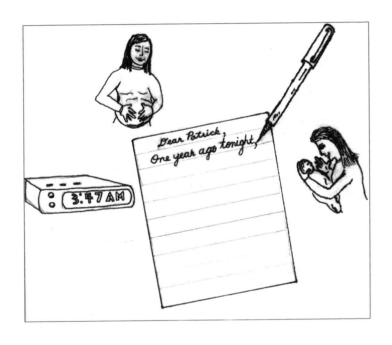

*Illustrated by Wendell E. Goff

Dear Patrick

By Angie Bolingbroke

One year ago tonight, you and I were one. You were not quite a person yet. I was already a mother one of one. I had spent 9 months loving, praying, dreaming, hoping, and wondering. As your arrival drew nearer, it was all over but the waiting. When would you come to greet us? I knew you so well! Those tiny feet that loved to kick right under my ribs, the midnight hiccups, and how you would protest when I ate Chinese food. You were so much a part of me.

And I wondered if you were figuring me out, too? Did you know of my love for you? Could you hear me then? The sound of my heart beating? The lullabies sung off key, but lovingly? Did those 9 months alone with me give you enough time to know how precious you are—at least enough to last until I can tell you again? I can only pray they did. And maybe we are now, as then, speaking truly heart to heart and soul to soul. For I have only my heart to speak to you—my hands haven't quite caught up.

One year ago tonight, I took a lot of things for granted. Too many things to list, really. Because of you, I no longer curse the steady ticking of the bathroom clock at 3:47 am on a sleepless night. And the whispered "I love you" as I tuck you in at night sometimes makes me wistful. Your sister's favorite lullaby had an entirely different meaning when I sing it to you—"You Are Very Special", in a way so completely different than she. The ease with which I toss about my words has sometimes become uncomfortable—because they are not yet shared with you. Do you, who a year ago was always included (by default), feel somehow excluded? I wonder if you wonder what you're missing. Or if you even know there's something to miss? I took communication for granted. Your first words. Your first sentence. I wondered how your little voice would sound, never dreaming the first time you said "Mommy" would be with hand to chin. You may never have funny ways to say "spaghetti" and "animal," but your cute little fingers will fumble in another version of baby-talk. And I promise I will celebrate and enjoy each one, mourning their passing as you master the language.

One year ago tonight, I thought I knew you, Patrick. But how could I know your infectious laugh, your sunny smile or your sparkling blue eyes? How could I guess at your always cheerful disposition? I knew you were stubborn, determined and ready for anything, but how could I know why you would need to be? Every day, I see more of you, of who you are and how much you have to teach me. What craziness for me to think I knew you so well that long year ago!

For you are so much more and better than I had imagined and because you are, so am I.

With love, Mommy

Angie Bolingbroke is a Virginia resident. She graduated from Pomona College with a BA in English Literature. Currently she is a domestic engineer, enjoying her time parenting her Deaf son, Patrick and his older sister, Katie.

When We Found Out

By Charlotte Wilhite

After 12 years of marriage and no children, major medical advances finally allowed us to conceive. After months of riding a rollercoaster of hope and depression, it finally paid off. Our son, Nick, was born to the most excited, loving, and prepared parents imaginable. He was our Golden Boy. We had such wonderful dreams for his future! We had read dozens of books so that we would be completely ready for our little boy. We had picked out his name when he was a thumb-sized fetus swimming around on the ultrasound screen. The whole pregnancy had gone wonderfully.

Mom was ecstatic; Dad was shyly proud; and every night we read to Nick while he was in the womb. We wanted him to know our voices. We let him listen to classical guitar, Beethoven, Rock 'n' Roll, and orchestra rehearsals. And as soon as we saw him, we both fell in love. I asked my mother on the phone that morning,

"Why didn't you tell me how wonderful babies are? Why didn't you tell me how much I would love him?"

She just sighed and giggled. "I tried, but you can't really tell someone how they will feel when they have a baby. New parents find out."

Every bit of those first 10 months was like heaven on earth. We loved watching him learn to smile, coo, kick his legs, and eat from a spoon. It was like a new romance. Then one day, he had a little cough. He woke up from his nap hot all over. The doctor did a lumbar puncture in her office. I was there and I saw the fluid. It was cloudy, like egg white.

"We need to get him admitted to the hospital, Charlotte," said the doctor. "It looks like meningitis."

Fear froze my heart. One of my high school friends had a son who died from meningitis at the age of 15 months.

"God," I prayed fervently, "You wouldn't take away my baby boy, would You? Not after so many years of praying for him, of waiting for him..."

Thoughts of Abraham and his son flickered through my mind. "You wouldn't take away my baby," I said with conviction.

We watched our baby helplessly as he lay passively in his hospital crib. His special blanket from home, his own stuffed toys, mobile of baby Shamus, and bunny music box were there with him to take away the gray starkness of the room.

Days of numbness, pain, and isolation followed. Max read medical books. It was his way of dealing with the stress of the situation. He quoted statistics: how many made it, how many died, the mortality and morbidity of the illness, the treatment options, the latest research.

Everything was done. I felt numb as I went through the familiar motions of caring for Nick in an unfamiliar place. Seizures sent him to the ICU. We were forced to leave during shift change and report time. It was the first time we'd had to leave our baby. He lay in a drug-induced coma attached to wires, tubes, and monitors. His skin seemed fragile, and his face looked as pale as a doll's.

Later that night, I was there alone with Nick. His nurse saw me sitting and looking at him. She asked, "Would you like to hold him?" My eyes lit up in surprise.

"Can I hold him with all those things attached to him?" I asked.

"Of course," replied the nurse. "We can move all the wires with him." She helped adjust the equipment and placed him in my arms. I held him the rest of the night as he slept.

The next day, Nick turned a corner. He started opening his eyes, looking around, and nursing! From there, he steadily progressed to trying to hold his head up (he was like a newborn baby) and moving his arms and legs. In the next few days, our little boy started trying to sit and stand, like he had done before, but he had no balance or strength. He didn't respond to his name anymore. The doctors told us that he might be deaf and could have seizures the rest of his life.

We didn't care a bit. He was our golden boy and he was going to make it. We could deal with the other stuff, no problem.

An ABR (Auditory Brainstem Response) was done before we left the hospital. This was a five-hour ordeal. They gave him drugs to sedate him, but it didn't work.

We held him, rocked him, sang to him, nursed him. Finally the results were there. The audiologist told us he had a hearing loss and explained the results. Then we took our baby home.

I remember feeling empty. We sat in the rocking chair where we had sat for months, and I had sung and read to him. The tapes he had enjoyed listening to, now lay next to the stereo. I didn't talk to him, and I didn't sing to him, and we didn't read. I didn't know what to do with him. I just held him, and weeks went by like that.

I looked in the yellow pages under "deaf." I had no idea where to start. We found a sign language class. We read books and found out how to interpret audiograms. Such sadness. Nick could not hear music anymore. Music had been a huge part of our lives. Max and I were both musical. We had grown up and met each other in a band.

We were part of a church singing group with an orchestra. We had a lifetime of memories surrounding music. Both of us played instruments and had paid our way through college with music scholarships. What would we do now? We could not share that with our son.

Even more frightening was the realization that we could not communicate. Nick no longer heard me when I talked to him. Before, I had kept up a running commentary (my husband will tell you I have the gift of gab):

"Okay, Nick, let's put on your shirt. Hold up your arms, good. Right hand, left hand, and over your head! Now the pants. Let's find your socks. Where are your shoes? You're such a cutie pie!"

I could no longer talk to him like this. How would I connect with him? How could I build a relationship, without the words?

Gradually, the answers began to come. Our doctor gave our number to another family with a deaf child, and the mother called me. What a wonderful feeling, knowing we weren't alone! And then, we started signing, very slowly and awkwardly.

More. Daddy. Drink. Finally, one day, our little baby boy signed back! More. Daddy. What a fabulous feeling! The joy was still there, because we still had our little boy.

We would never pretend that it is all is smooth sailing. We revisit times of grief over and over in our lives. The first time we saw him with hearing aids on. Watching other children his age, talking with their parents and their little friends. Seeing my sister read effortlessly to her children with them snuggled on her lap and beside her. Hearing my little nieces use words like "crouton" or "broccoli"; words that we knew no signs for. Seeing Nick compensate for lack of language by kicking or biting or tantrums. Realizing that most of his family will never know him as we do. Wishing we could share the beauty of English literature and poetry and music.

Three years after Nick was in the ICU, I was in nursing school doing pediatric clinical rotations at the same children's hospital. My face was hot and my heart raced as I waited to go on an ICU tour with my fellow nursing students. I stared at the floor, thinking, "I can do this. Nick is not in there now. He is OK. We have moved on."

Then one of my nursing friends, who knew about Nick, asked me gently:

"Are you thinking about your little boy?"

I burst into soul-wrenching sobs and fled down the hallway to escape the memory of that place where my son had lain so still and pale three years before. My instructor came to find me. She put her arms around me and let me finish crying. After I calmed down, she said, "It's okay. You don't have to go in there again... you don't have to go."

The times of pain are becoming less frequent. There are times of revelation, learning, and hope. We realize these things when we meet Deaf adults whom we admire and respect. When Nick learns how to play a new game, asks a thoughtful question, or tells a funny story. When we see other children who have more severe disabilities but still struggle on. And when someone else understands.

I am now a pediatric nurse. Isn't that funny? My instructor thought it was, when she saw me a few years later. We had a laugh about it and I told her,

"I was drawn to pediatrics because of my personal experience with my child. I feel that I am a much better nurse because of it. I know what those parents are going through. I can meet their needs better because I understand."

Whenever I see a parent sitting at the bedside of their sick child, I ask them if they would like to hold him. The gratitude on the parent's face gives me such heart-warming satisfaction. And I understand.

Charlotte Wilhite is a registered nurse, part time-interpreter and has had several photographs published in *Memory Maker's Magazine*. She lives with her husband Max and their nine-year-old son, Nick, in Ft. Worth, Texas. Nick lost his hearing after contracting meningitis at age 10 months.

My Deafness is...So What?

By Mary Jane Rhodes

My son, Ronnie, attended the Indiana School for the Deaf as a child. He was involved in many activities at school, especially athletics. One year he earned letters in football, basketball, baseball, wrestling and track; the next year he added swimming to the list. My husband Joe and I always made an effort to see all of his games and other athletic events. At ISD, parents were often involved in activities at the school. Our social life has always involved parents of other Deaf children who were attending the Indiana School.

One of our disappointments, however, was finding so few Deaf people in various jobs and professional positions. We realized how important it was for Deaf children to have Deaf role models. It seemed to us that there was a desperate need for Deaf social workers, preachers, psychologists, educators and vocational rehabilitation counselors. So in one of my "From A Parent's Point of View" columns that appeared in *The Deaf American* magazine, I made the following plea to the Deaf community:

"I love my son and am proud of him. It is because of this love for him and pride in him that I can acknowledge that I now need your help. Surely there must be untapped reservoirs of talented and capable leaders among your ranks. Will you men and women who live in the world of the Deaf, please find the courage to step forward and insist on filling positions of leadership that are now, and will, become available?

Would you take my son's hand and lead him... and if God be willing, can you please show him how to use his leadership abilities, so that some day he can also guide other Deaf children over the bumps and around the curves that they encounter in their silent world? I realize I am asking a lot from the Deaf citizens of the United States — but I am asking so much, only because I feel confident that you have much to give."

An answer to my plea came on November 14, 1968, when Ronnie and I were invited to participate in the Midwestern Regional Deaf Youth Leadership Demonstration. High school aged Deaf students from twenty-four schools, representing nineteen states and the District of Columbia, confirmed my belief in the great potential of our Deaf youth. How exciting it was to see evidence of leadership abilities among these Junior National Association of the Deaf members!

During this event, the young leaders from each school interacted with adult Deaf leaders. These men and women represented the National Association of the Deaf, the Council of Organizations Serving the Deaf, the Registry of Interpreters for the Deaf, the National Theater of the Deaf, the National Technical Institute for the Deaf, Gallaudet College, the Professional Rehabilitation Workers with the Adult Deaf, the National Fraternal Society of the Deaf, the Indiana Association of the Deaf, and several other organizations.

Cathy Monroe, first runner-up for Miss America 1969, was an immediate hit with the Junior NAD. She had performed a song in sign language on national television as her talent contribution, which was a giant breakthrough for Deaf citizens. For Cathy to use sign language as a creative art form during a time when Deaf children were still being punished for signing was a great morale builder for the national Deaf community. As might be expected, we all loved having Cathy with us.

I longed for other moms and dads to share my experience as I mingled with the other participants. If parents who felt their Deaf sons and daughters were doomed to an unhappy and unproductive life could see these Junior NAD students, they would gain a different perspective about deafness. Deaf adult leaders were sharing their accomplishments, motivating Deaf students to assume new roles of leadership for the future. The students were urged to look at their deafness as an inconvenience, not a handicap. "You have much to contribute to your own communities, your state and your nation," they were told.

It was exciting for me to see the lives and accomplishments of so many Deaf leaders. I was sure that if other parents of Deaf children could see and understand this, they would become more fully involved in their children's world of silence. But sadly, the controversy over methods of communication robbed many parents of the opportunity to share and participate in the lives of Deaf adults. The stigma against sign language drove a wedge between them and all Deaf people, not just their own sons and daughters. If parents would accept sign language, much of the burden of communication and their children's deafness could be lifted from their hearts.

The battle over communication methods had become tiresome and we decided to do something about it once and for all. There was some talk about making Deaf Power a slogan and rallying cry for Deaf Americans, but instead we decided to go with Deaf Pride. With Deaf Pride would come Deaf Power and the potential to grow. The emphasis on Deaf Pride would bring opportunity and acceptance, whereas Deaf Power might have suggested a belligerent attitude. It was Deaf Pride that would bring forth many positive and mighty changes.

I had some buttons produced to help launch Deaf Pride, and in the months to follow there were thousands of Deaf youth and adults wearing their Deaf Pride buttons. Thousands more hearing parents and friends joined in, making Deaf Pride visible across the nation.

With all of the emphasis on Deaf youth preparing themselves for roles of leadership, Ronnie came home one evening to announce that he decided to become a psychologist. This was exciting news. Deaf professionals trained to serve the Deaf population were critically needed, and I complimented Ronnie on his decision. About a month later, I asked him if he still planned to become a psychologist. Ronnie had a way of looking at life that always seemed to produce an unexpected twist. So I couldn't help laughing when, with a hint of a grin, he said: "No, I have decided not to become a psychologist. I am afraid that all of that studying might damage my brain."

Meanwhile, I was invited to assist in planning the first National Association of the Deaf Youth Leadership Camp. One snowy night in February, we arrived in Stroudsburg, Pennsylvania, where twelve men, eleven of them Deaf, welcomed me. Everyone there had traveled considerable distances through the inclement weather to lend their time and talent to build the next generation of Deaf leaders. God was blessing me greatly, by permitting me to have an inside view of my son's world.

In April of 1969, I traveled to Texas to take part in the Youth Leadership Demonstration at the Texas School for the Deaf. I chaperoned Ronnie and several other representatives from the Indiana School, and we brought an unusual prop, a broom. The broom was part of the message the Indiana Junior NAD members spread among their Texas cohorts, urging them to "sweep away the barriers of Deafness."

On our way to Texas, we stopped in Memphis to change flights. Before we boarded the next plane, I realized I had left the broom on the first flight, and I went to retrieve it. Upon returning to the terminal, I was surprised to find all of my students gathered around a man. It was Dr. Pete Merrill, who had just been elected to become the new President at Gallaudet College. Dr. Merrill was to make valuable and innovative changes in the course of Gallaudet College, the only college for Deaf students in the world (later to become Gallaudet University). It was so inspiring to see Dr. Merrill caught up in the excitement of Deaf youth who were just starting to spread their wings.

Upon arriving at the Texas School and participating in group discussions, I was surprised to see how knowledgeable our Deaf youth had become. They understood the educational retardation forced upon deaf students by oralism. Some commented on the necessity for improved social adjustment, while others focused on their desire for family members to accept them as equals. These young students had definite ideas about the need for parent education, improved vocational opportunities and how their schools could better serve Deaf students. Ronnie loved this experience and the chance to exchange ideas with Deaf peers from all over the country. He also took advantage of the opportunity to discuss these issues with adult Deaf leaders, who came to share their hopes and dreams with the Deaf leaders of the future.

Not long after the Texas Youth Leadership Demonstration, Ronnie was excited to find that he was one of the students invited to apply for the Junior NAD Leadership Camp in Pennsylvania. Students interested in attending had to write an essay on why they wanted to participate, and Ronnie had spent several hours preparing his entry. When he finished his essay, he handed it over to me for feedback. It looked good and he had done all the work himself, but I found a few parts that could have used some corrections in punctuation or sentence structure. I picked up a pencil and began to make a few notations on the paper when Ronnie, who was watching closely, stopped me. "I don't want you to change what I wrote," he explained. He was only looking for some general feedback, emphasizing "I want my ideas in there, not yours!" Ronnie was absolutely right. Hearing people had been telling Deaf students how to think for far too long. I left his paper as it was, and his essay won the right to participate in the camp.

Shortly afterwards, I was invited to join my son for a week at the Junior NAD Leadership Camp. During my stay, I did a survey of the campers. One question was related to what jobs they hoped to have in the future. Nineteen out of thirty-seven indicated they wanted to become teachers. Others expressed interest in becoming an author, a harness racing jockey, an aerospace engineer, an oceanography photographer, a social worker, a counselor, a missionary, a politician, a computer programmer, a printer, and an entrepreneur.

These were impressive goals for a generation of Deaf youth who had been raised in a world that generally ignored them and their dreams of tomorrow. This kind of positive thinking reminded me of the time Ronnie had come in to announce how he planned to enter the Deaf Olympics. Having just discovered that International Olympics for the Deaf were held every four years, he didn't want to miss the action. When I expressed my delight and asked him what event he planned to compete in, he replied, "Oh, I haven't decided yet!" He felt sure he could accomplish his goal of being in the Olympics regardless, and this kind of positive thinking was evident in all of the young Deaf campers.

Another question the survey asked for was a suggestion on how parents could help their Deaf children. A large majority of the campers expressed their desire for parents to learn sign language. There was a suggestion that parents should explain to strangers that their child is Deaf. Another asked parents to interpret television and radio programs as well as other hearing peoples' conversations. Several felt their moms and dads overprotected them, and asked parents to trust them and believe in their ability to do things. One youth said, "Don't worry so much about your Deaf child. Let him do everything the other children in the family do." Well said!

Associating with these Deaf campers and their adult Deaf role models confirmed my belief that every deaf person in the country has a right to Deaf Pride. Certainly, Deaf people should not be made to feel ashamed of their deafness. Yet, by forcing them to use only speech and speechreading, we have done exactly that. Many Deaf students over the years were led to believe that unless they could become proficient at oral communication, they were failures. The fact that only a small percentage of prelingual Deaf students were able to become adept at speech destined most of the Deaf population to second-class citizenship.

In spite of the persecution that a majority of our Deaf students were subject to, many of the men who helped plan the Leadership Camp went on to earn their doctorates. Dr. Robert Davilla was in this group of Deaf men, and he later became the Assistant Secretary for the Office of Special Education and Rehabilitation Services in the U.S.

Department of Education. Many of the youth who attended the camp have also, one way or the other, become leaders in today's national Deaf community.

Finally, there was another touching moment which came out of the survey I conducted at the Camp. I was reading responses to the question, "What are your feelings about being Deaf?" My heart rejoiced as I read the following answers:

"I am proud that I am Deaf. Also, I'm glad that God gave it to me."

"I am proud that I am me; I do not care if I am Deaf or not."

"I am proud since I am as happy as I can be."

"I've no bad thoughts about Deafness. I just feel proud that I am Deaf."

"I don't feel ashamed. I want to be proud that I am Deaf and show the hearing people that I can do as they do."

As I sorted through these answers, I came across a familiar-looking piece of writing. Upon taking a closer look, I realized it was Ronnie's handwriting. And true to his nature, he had this very positive response towards his Deafness:

"I am really proud to be Deaf," he wrote. "I don't want to be a hearing person. My Deafness is... SO WHAT!"

Mary Jane Rhodes is currently the editor of *Deaf Fellowship for Jesus* Newsletter. She has written for *The Deaf American, New Jersey Speech & Hearing Association Journal* and many other publications.

Ron Rhodes is now a teacher at the School for the Deaf in Fremont, California. He has been the President of the Deaf Counseling and Referral Agency (DCARA) in the San Francisco Bay area and has served three terms as the President of the California Association of the Deaf. His Jr. NAD Leadership Training helped prepare him for the contributions he is making as a leader in the Deaf Community today.

Deaf Community And Technology:

A Love-Hate Relationship

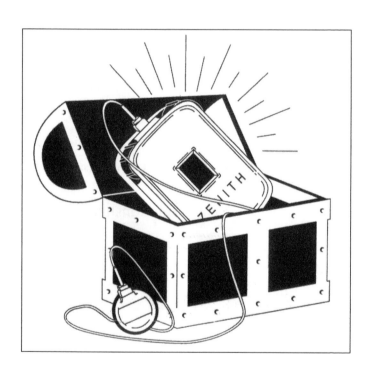

*Illustrated by Lois A. Lehman-Lenderman

Good Luck Charm Hearing Aid

By Lois A. Lehman-Lenderman

You might have heard of (or perhaps used) a rabbit's foot as a good luck charm. But have you heard of a hearing aid bringing luck? Let me tell a tale about mine.

In 1974, my Deaf older sister, Anita and her ex-husband, Bob, cleaned the storage room and found his old hearing aid. He laughed about finding it because he had refused to wear it at school as a teenager. He was never comfortable with it. When he opened the battery lid, he was shocked to see my name etched in the metal lid. Anita thought he had taken it from me by mistake during my summer stay with them in early 1970's, but he swore it was the one his parents bought him.

My school, Iowa School for the Deaf, and his school, the Nebraska School for the Deaf in Omaha, are only eleven miles apart. Apparently in the early 1960's, when I was little and received a new hearing aid, my school audiologist forgot to etch out my name on the hearing aid case before she passed it on to Bob's school audiologist. It was then given to Bob. All this time, Bob was unaware of my name in his hearing aid –and he went on to marry my sister in 1966.

Unfortunately, this lucky charm didn't last forever. Bob and Anita, who had two sons together, divorced in the late 1970's (Anita is currently married to LaWayne Beery). Nonetheless, that hearing aid made an unusual connection, and perhaps we should remember it as a hearing aid-in-law.

Lois A. Lehman-Lenderman graduated from the Iowa School for the Deaf in 1971 and received her Bachelor Degree in Art from Gallaudet University in 1976. She is married to Bob Lenderman and currently works as an illustrator for the United States Air Force Headquarters at the Pentagon in Washington, DC.

Technology and the Deaf

By Bonnie E. Thomas
(as told to Mark Drolsbaugh)

Someone recently asked me an intriguing question: how has your life changed as a result of the new technology that is now available to the Deaf and hard of hearing? Tremendously, of course. But to truly show the impact it's had, I need to give you some background on what it was like growing up before technological advances came into my life.

I was born Deaf. However, Deafness wasn't acceptable in my family. I wasn't allowed to associate with my grandfather's brother, who was also Deaf. My grandfather and I were close, but he was forbidden to use sign language in my presence. Such was the environment that I grew in; I had to be shielded from anything related to Deaf Culture.

Nonetheless, in 1990, I found out about the strong Deaf community and became a part of it. In a way, I was born again, born into the Deaf world. Previously, because I'd been pressured to conform to hearing values, I would always pretend to understand what hearing people were saying. It was a hearing world, and I needed to fit in as best as I could.

There were limits to how well I could bluff my way through spoken conversations with hearing people. At hearing social events, I could always be found in the kitchen; it was tiresome to socialize because of the limited conversation available to someone who can't hear.

As a Deaf person, on the other hand, I've become very productive. I could never imagine returning to the passive existence of trying to blend in with the hearing world.

Prior to 1990, I knew no sign language and knew nothing about the various technologies that were available to the Deaf. Little did I know that all of the accessibility technology that had been developed would become a lifeline for me and the rest of the Deaf community.

And so, we come to how my life has changed because of technology. How has it changed, you ask? Let me count the ways!

I have no idea how I lived all these years without closed-captioned TV. I got my first taste of captioned television in 1990. I am grateful to the Nickleodeon channel, because they have captioned many of the old classic shows that I missed while growing up! I'm so happy to have finally caught up with all of the popular shows that are on today. Some improvements are needed in areas such as real-time captioning, like when regular shows are interrupted with late breaking news reports. Overall, I feel that watching television is a whole lot more enjoyable and educational than ever before.

Moving on... oh, how I love my TTY. Really! I lived in complete denial of being Deaf for so many years, insisting on speaking by voice on the phone (obviously, not so easy to do when you're Deaf). When I finally came to terms with my Deafness, the first thing I purchased was a TTY. A friend had demonstrated it for me. I will never forget the first time I used it. It was amazing to be able to understand every single word for the first time in my life. I would never have to struggle with a phone conversation again.

Not everyone I call has a TTY, but that's where the Relay Service comes in. A number of Deaf and hearing people have complained about it for one reason or another, but I think it's a fabulous service! Sometimes we forget what life was like before this service was available. I used to have to drive to various offices to make appointments for myself. I remember the first time I ordered a pizza delivery through the relay (the New Jersey Relay Service premiered in 1991). It is such a godsend, and has made life much easier in so many ways.

E-mail is fast becoming the ultimate lifeline for Deaf people! If you have America Online, it's really mind-blowing! With AOL you can use chat rooms or instant messaging to visit online with friends and others in real time. Deaf people usually feel isolated during the time between Deaf events and gatherings; with e-mail and online services, we can keep in touch with more people, more conveniently. It doesn't cost extra to chat using instant messages or chat rooms, and several of your friends can join in on the conversation. If we did this by TTY, my phone bill would go through the roof. I have never had so much contact with so many people, until I got online services. I got my first personal computer in 1997, and my life has improved incredibly since then.

Open-captioned movies were introduced in New Jersey not too long ago, as the technology became available in May of 1998. The first captioned film I ever attended at a movie theater was *Titanic*. It was absolutely wonderful to be able to attend such a popular event! The only limitation is that most places offering open-captioned movies only schedule them for once a month and for one showing only. I still don't have the freedom to go and catch a movie anytime I please. Perhaps by the year 2025 or so, I guess.

I don't mean to sound pessimistic, but it depresses me when Deaf people are treated like second class citizens. Don't get me wrong, I do appreciate the hard work and effort it took to make open-captioned movies a reality. It's just that when we only have one movie captioned on one specific day at one specific time in one specific theater, it's like we're being shuffled off into some remote corner. And the movies chosen aren't always blockbusters like *Titanic*; sometimes we get box office flops while the hearing world has unlimited access to all the best films. Again, this is a very new service and there's still room for improvement, but it's a step in the right direction. It will probably get better. For now, we will just rent captioned videotapes as the new releases come out.

My pager is invaluable. I have an alphanumeric pager that I'm very satisfied with. People can page me using a TTY number, a voice dispatcher, or even AOL (which has a setup that allows pages to be sent if one has a program called MobileComm). And no, this is not any ordinary pager that just gives callback numbers; it sends and receives messages that provide important information. Numerous Deaf professionals have benefited from having these pagers in many situations, especially in emergencies.

Traveling and staying in hotels is a new experience now. A number of hotels are now in compliance with the ADA (Americans with Disabilities Act) laws. They provide TTYs, and assistive devices such as flashing lights, which alert me to someone knocking on the door or an alarm going off, as well as built-in captioning on the televisions. Some hotels accessibility-ready upon check-in, while others provide what is called an ADA kit. This isn't the easiest thing to manage. It's a heavy suitcase loaded with all of the accessible equipment, which you often have to haul up to your room and set up yourself! Can you imagine hearing people checking into a hotel, and having to install the phones, televisions, alarm clocks, and fire alarms? That's how absurd it feels when Deaf people are handed an ADA kit.

Ultimately, the best experience I ever had staying at a hotel was at none other than Gallaudet University, in the Kellogg Conference Center. Everyone at the front desk, Deaf or non-Deaf, uses sign language. Every room is fully accessible. The whole building is Deaf-friendly in every aspect. With one visit there, I realized what it's like for a hearing person to be able to walk into a hotel and experience total comfort and convenience. The Kellogg Conference Center sets the standard other hotels need to strive for when it comes to ADA compliance.

Well, there you have it. There have been a lot of improvements in accessibility for the Deaf community. Just imagining what life was like beforehand is comparison enough; we've truly come a long way. But it actually goes deeper than that. When you factor in my former life, when I was trying to do things the hearing way, and the frustrations that came with it, then the recent technological advances in become all the more meaningful. Today, I truly enjoy life on my terms, as a Deaf person.

Bonnie E. Thomas was born and raised in New York and currently resides in Bergen County, NJ. Bonnie is very involved with the NJ Deaf Community, particularly with setting up events for Deaf children.

Unusual Interview

By Michael Callejas

It was not long after graduating from college that I began a concentrated effort at job-hunting. Employment agencies, organizations serving the deaf, the classified pages... you name it, I tried it.

One of the places I went to was the Employment Resource Center downtown. I copied pages from books advertising civil job openings, looking for jobs that matched my qualifications, and then I sent in countless resumes.

After the first week went by with no response, I wasn't too worried. These things take time. When the second week passed, I reassured myself that no one really finds a job that fast. When the third week passed, I began to get anxious.

I couldn't believe it! No one had called or written. Not a peep. I thought I'd done everything right, and that if I job hunted aggressively, I'd see results quickly. It just wasn't happening. I had to give myself a pep talk.

"Have patience," I said. "Sooner or later, a call or letter has to come in. Someone eventually has to notice what I have to offer!"

Another month had passed with no response. I knew job hunting wasn't easy, but this was getting ridiculous. My patience was sorely tested. Naturally, I began to feel a bit discouraged.

Still, I pressed on. Not having a source of income is a powerful motivation to keep searching for a job. It also helped that I had my own team of cheerleaders: parents, siblings, and friends. They would not let me give up, and were always offering encouragement.

With renewed energy, I threw myself into the job hunt once again. By the second month, I actually began to receive correspondence from various companies— in the form of rejection letters. This put such a damper on my efforts that I started to question if I was sufficiently educated or experienced to do anything. Was there a job out there at all for me? Anything?

When my mother heard of my desperation, she secretly told my relatives and friends about my frustrations. Without my knowledge, she asked them if they knew of anyone who needed a junior accountant or administrative assistant.

By the end the third month of my job search, my Aunt Mary called me via the California Relay Service. She invited me over to her house, and I gladly went because it gave me a chance to see her and my favorite hearing cousins. Besides, at this point, I had nothing else to do.

Aunt Mary and I had a pleasant talk. Then, out of the blue, she told me she had a friend who needed a temporary employee. She explained that it was an accounting job, which seemed like a perfect fit, as this was my college major. The opportunity was at the Hyatt Hotel, at Fisherman's Wharf.

Initially, I hesitated because it was only a temporary job, but then I realized that beggars couldn't be choosers. I decided to take her friend up on the offer. If nothing else, it would add experience to my resume and help me land another job someday. I told Aunt Mary to call her friend and let her know that I was interested. Shortly afterwards, Aunt Mary's friend returned the call, and we set up an interview for August fifth. At last! Things were starting to look up. I couldn't wait!

When August fifth rolled around, I showed up at the Hyatt Hotel, eager to begin the interview. I gave the receptionist a short note that stated my name and objective, a job interview with the Human Resource Manager. She called her supervisor, who instructed her to take me up to the office.

While the receptionist led me upstairs, I began to put pressure on myself. I knew I needed to make a strong first impression. I <u>had</u> to ace this interview. I knew I could do it. I would impress the interviewer so much that she would offer me the job on the spot. Or would she? Perhaps with my luck, I'd botch everything and get thrown out the door. No, no, I couldn't allow myself to think that way. I had to think positively.

Prior to entering the manager's office, I gave myself a pep talk to get my confidence back — but my optimism vanished the minute I entered the manager's office. For right there, at that very moment, I suddenly realized an incredible oversight. *I had not requested an interpreter for the interview!*

At this juncture, my palms were getting sweaty! I made an effort to keep smiling. The manager, Miss Kendricks, was a friendly, attractive blonde who stood up as soon as I entered her office. Smiling politely, she apparently said,

"Hi I'm Anne Kendricks. Nice to meet you."

At least that's what I think she said. It was hard to read her lips. I'm not a skilled lipreader, so I could only guess what she was saying and try to fill in the blanks. All I could do was nod my head and smile.

Miss Kendricks then extended her hand and I followed suit. We shook hands politely.

With that out of the way, she began to fire questions at me.

"Okay here goes," I thought, "It's time to let the cat out of the bag."

I gathered up all my courage and gestured that I couldn't hear. At first, Miss Kendricks looked puzzled and asked me another question. I repeated the gesture. Then an odd expression came over Miss Kendrick's face as she realized that I couldn't hear, or verbally respond to, her questions. She was absolutely stunned, and gestured for me to sit down. Then she sat down to try to make sense of this.

We were both stumped on how to communicate at first, but I quickly recovered and gestured that I needed paper and a pen. She obliged, and we began a second attempt at our interview.

Within five minutes, Miss Kendricks had a new idea. She gestured "wait" by raising her palm up. She got up and approached the bookshelves behind her desk. After digging around for a while, she bent down and picked something up. To my surprise, it was a TTY. Grabbing the paper and pen we were using, she wrote,

"I don't remember how to set this up...can you do it for me?"

I nodded happily. I plugged it into the socket and typed, "Hello, I'm Michael Callejas. Shall we start the interview all over again?"

"Gladly," was her typed reply.

After a half-hour interview via TTY, Miss Kendricks offered me the position.

"Mr. Callejas," she remarked, "I must confess that this was the most unusual interview I've ever conducted. But it was not at all the unpleasant experience I anticipated."

I looked up at her face and saw a broad smile that radiated sincere warmth. Needless to say, as soon as I saw her smile, I knew I had the job. All of the obstacles and frustrations that I had encountered had become irrelevant. Unusual interview or not, we had improvised, and accomplished our goal.

Michael Callejas currently lives in California and works as a library assistant. He is an avid collector of comic books.

Our Cochlear Implant Decision

By Charlotte Wilhite

I know it's a touchy subject and everyone has their own ideas about it. I'm talking about the cochlear implant. There are so many opinions, good and bad, about this intriguing yet controversial technology. I would like to make this clear: it is not my intention to judge anyone's family or decisions regarding the cochlear implant. I would not question it any more than I would question a person's choice of religion. All I intend to do is share my personal experience, acknowledging the difficult process involved in making such a decision.

My son Nick was ten months old when he lost his hearing to meningitis. That was about eight years ago. At the time, my husband Max and I had no idea how much hearing was lost. It's quite difficult to determine with a baby.

By the time Nick was two years old, we saw a doctor to determine if he might be a candidate for a cochlear implant. This was just part of our never-ending search for information and wisdom regarding the choices we make for our family.

The doctor, without so much as a second glance at Nick's chart, asked us what we thought our son could hear.

"Well, he doesn't hear much," I explained. "Dogs barking, thunder, balloons popping, big trucks... that's about it."

"If I were you," the doctor intoned, "I would insist on a cochlear implant for him." We were a bit taken aback. We asked the doctor why he felt that way.

"Because," he continued, " if you ever want him to hear and speak, that's what you need to do."

"But what about the risks," I asked. "Possible infection, facial nerve paralysis, death under anesthesia? Can you say without a doubt that the benefits outweigh the risks?"

"Of course I can't," the doctor hedged. "You know, there are no guarantees. The cochlear implant may not work for everyone. And it's only recently been approved for use in children, but your son would be followed by researchers with much interest, and there would be hardly any cost to you."

"Cost is not an issue," I said. "What about the risks?"

"Oh, the surgery is really simple," the doctor assured. "Of course, sometimes there are complications, but they're rare. If you ever want your son to be normal, then you should have the implant done."

"That's easy for you to say," I replied. "It isn't your child's life at stake. You get paid quite well for the surgery and have little to lose."

"Well, that's a little harsh," said the doctor. "Of course, I have my patients' best interests at heart."

"Yes, I'm sorry, we know you do." I felt awkward challenging the doctor, but I was still somewhat hesitant about the implant. "It's just that you don't have much to lose, and we have everything to lose. Perhaps we could wait a while and see how other children are doing with the implant?"

"The time is now if you want to do this," the doctor insisted. "The benefits of doing it later will be less than the benefits of getting it done now. When Nick gets older, he may forget any sounds he heard during his first ten months."

"But, in a few years, there may be more advances in cochlear implant technology," I countered.

"I don't think so. If any advances are made, they will be in the processor, not in the implant." The doctor was still pressuring us.

"But would we have to give up sign language and start over from the beginning with the oral method?" I asked.

"Most children with implants," the doctor explained, "need an oral-auditory approach. Sign language isn't going to enhance oral and auditory skills."

"But he already knows several hundred words in sign language," I protested. "We can communicate freely with him. And if something were to happen to his facial nerve... he needs facial expressions to communicate! His facial expressions are what give him his charm and help him connect with other people. We can't risk the loss of that for anything!"

"It is only a small risk," the doctor reassured me. "But if you ever expect him to integrate into American culture, this is the only way to do it."

Max and I left the doctor's office with an uneasy feeling. We didn't feel comfortable with the idea of implanting our son. We had met with other parents of children who had gotten implants, and their stories were different from ours. Almost all of the success stories had been about children who were already talking when they lost their hearing. One or two had a progressive loss and did not become profoundly deaf until they were eight or nine years old, when English was already firmly established in their language base. The parents described how, prior to the implant, these children had been left out of social activities, which had left them withdrawn and unhappy.

Apparently, these postlingual deaf children wanted to talk, but were frustrated in their efforts to do so. After getting the cochlear implant, their lives had changed for the better. They were happier, more outgoing and confident, and participated in family and school life to a greater extent.

Our child, however, wasn't withdrawn. He was happy just as he was. He didn't seem to be frustrated by his inability to speak. He seemed perfectly normal to us. We decided to ask him what he thought, even though he was only two years old at the time.

"Nick," I began. "If you had the chance to hear... if something could be put inside your head and you could hear people talking... music... trucks... would you want to have that?"

"Mmmm..." Nick replied. "I would like to hear trucks."

We thought about it some more. There was not enough research out there about cochlear implants being used on very young, prelingual deaf children. There were no promises or even probabilities that the implant would work for our child.

I thought about a boy I had spoken with at a cochlear implant group meeting, a boy who had received the implant when he was nine years old. We had been in a crowded room with several other people talking, but he was able to understand almost everything I said. I felt that I had to ask him a personal question.

"How old were you when you became Deaf?" I asked.

"What do you mean?" he replied.

"When did you become Deaf?"

"I'm not Deaf." He looked a bit confused. "I've never been Deaf."

We conversed some more, and I asked him about his daily life with the implant. I wanted to know whether he could hear using only his hearing aid on the other ear, whether he could hear with the implant alone, and whether he could participate in sports. His answer to all of my questions was, yes. I also wanted to know if he knew any sign language.

"I'm learning sign language in case I ever need it," he replied.

Some children we met had the implant, but didn't use it anymore. These kids did not attend the aforementioned cochlear implant meetings, but I felt I needed to seek them out because I wanted to understand as many perspectives as possible.

One boy, a fifth grader at Nick's school, walked around with his implant receiver hanging from his ear. His teacher explained that she tried to encourage him to use it, but that he took it off as often as he could. The teacher remarked that she didn't think he got much benefit from it, anyway.

There was another boy whose family had invested a lot of time and energy into his cochlear implant. They sadly acknowledged that it didn't seem to help. The boy's lipreading seemed to improve, but "He didn't hear or talk any better than before," his parents noted. They wondered out loud if his lipreading skills would have improved anyway, without the implant.

Two other children I knew, each with major developmental delays, underwent surgery for cochlear implants. I could not see any benefit in either case. When I looked into their faces, they barely made eye contact. They ignored me when I talked or signed to them. One seemed to look right through me. I couldn't understand how the cochlear implant was helping her.

All of the children I knew with a cochlear implant had it put in for free, so cost was never really a concern. As Nick's doctor had mentioned, there were plenty of researchers who, at the time, were excited about the new technology. They wanted more children to participate in their studies. All of the surgical procedures and costs were covered by the companies involved (and perhaps some of our tax dollars). The bottom line was that none of the families had to pay anything, regardless of their incomes.

For the next year or so, Max and I talked with different families, as well as various professionals who worked with cochlear implants. We read all the literature we could get our hands on. Most of the printed material at that time was published by the cochlear implant industry, so although the information was clear and informative, we felt there was no way it could be completely unbiased.

We began to feel that the perfect cochlear implant recipient would be a child who had learned his family's spoken language already, and then suddenly or progressively lost his hearing. Most children in this category did exceptionally well with implants. They only had to re-learn what the sounds they were receiving meant. They already had developed a language to form an association between sounds and meaning. We had never met a prelingual Deaf child who had received the implant and was now talking and hearing with it (Note: this was at a time when there were very few prelingual Deaf children with the implant who had reached four years of age).

We also noticed that for some reason, the Deaf community was outraged by the implanting of young children. We tried to understand their point of view, visiting with many Deaf adults and listening to them explain why they felt the way that they did.

One lady told us she had seen a young girl with an incision on her head. Among her comments: "I felt such sadness that they would put a foreign object into a baby like that. Such a big scar! And it won't make her hearing. The parents are just in denial that their daughter is Deaf."

I considered that. A big scar didn't worry me. I am a nurse and I know that in virtually all surgeries, there will be a scar. The impact on a person's life isn't measured by the size of a scar that will be under his or her hair, anyway. Granted, for many people the thought of someone's head being cut open and their skull being drilled into is very frightening. But, I knew that the surgical procedure itself would not be the deciding factor for our family (all surgical risks notwithstanding).

What concerned me the most was the comment about parents being in denial. We knew that denial was a normal part of the grieving process. Were we in denial? We didn't feel like we were. We had accepted our son completely, hadn't we? If he had needed, say, an eye prosthesis or a kidney transplant, we wouldn't have hesitated.

My Deaf friends vehemently insisted that a kidney transplant was much different; in that scenario, it's a matter of life and death. With deafness, however, a person could live a perfectly normal, happy life. Arguably, there was nothing abnormal or incomplete about being Deaf.

"I would hate it if my parents had done that to me," most of my Deaf friends said. Almost all of them knew of a Deaf adult who had the implant but didn't use it. I was absolutely mystified at the strength of opposition coming from the Deaf community. I couldn't understand why they would object so strongly, because certainly some children might be able to benefit from having the implant.

I read a pamphlet circulated by the local Deaf community. It was not entirely accurate. The pamphlet claimed that people with cochlear implants couldn't play sports, for example. I knew for a fact that was false. Another argument in the pamphlet was that a person with the implant would not be able to undergo Magnetic Resonance Imaging (MRI). Well, I wasn't worried about my child not having MRIs. There are plenty of other diagnostic procedures, and besides, a newer version of the cochlear implant would allow for MRIs.

Reading further into the pamphlet, it decried how parents were being deceived into thinking their children would become hearing. Wanting so badly for their children to be hearing like themselves, parents were making uninformed, emotional decisions that they had no right to make for a potential member of the Deaf community.

Even though I saw a grain of truth in this statement, it angered me. I felt that parents were guilty of nothing more than loving their children and wanting what's best for them. Is that so bad? Deaf children of hearing parents do not, in my opinion, "belong" to the Deaf community. My child belongs to my family.

Philosophical and emotional issues notwithstanding, my husband was more concerned about the benefits to risk ratio. He didn't want our son undergoing any surgical procedure, unless there was a reasonably high probability that it would make a positive difference in his life. I agreed, all the while listening to a tiny voice inside me, a gut feeling which kept telling me that the cochlear implant would not be right for my son.

I tried to imagine Nick as an adult, making the decision for himself. I listened as hard as I could for what he might be feeling. I thought about my Deaf adult friends who had shared their feelings with me. I wondered again if I was indeed going through some sort of denial regarding Nick's hearing loss. I wondered, "What if we got Nick the implant? Suppose it didn't work and it destroyed his facial nerve?" I also wondered if perhaps the implant was an ideal option for Nick, and that we were making a mistake by waiting too long. Perhaps it would be too late if we waited any longer.

When Nick was three years old, we traveled to a larger city in our region and consulted with a different doctor (who had also performed the cochlear implant procedure) for a second opinion. We had sent Nick's audiograms, medical history and a thorough description of his hearing ability to the doctor's office two weeks in advance. Upon meeting him in person, we inquired some more, sharing our concerns with him.

This doctor was more guarded in his reply than the one we had seen before. He appeared to be more neutral and up front about the risks.

"It is indeed a surgery with risks," the doctor explained. "The facial nerve lies very near the auditory nerve. We are getting some good reports back from the research, but it is too soon to tell if your son will have any benefit."

"Doctor," I asked, "What do you make of the Deaf community's strong negative reaction to the cochlear implant?"

"Well, they are certainly entitled to their opinions. But I don't think most of them are very well informed. The implant has improved quite a bit since it was first introduced. Regardless, this is your decision to make and you have to consider what is best for your child."

We left this doctor's office in a confident state of mind. We were Nick's parents, and after all, the Lord must have known what he was doing when he gave Nick to us. We were competent, and we had the right to make the decision ourselves.

That night, I asked Nick again: "If there were something that could help you hear, would you want it?"

He was interested, and this time around, he was able to ask more questions. I tried to downplay the surgery part, knowing that aspect would frighten him. However, Nick's response was notably different from before.

"I don't know..." he said. "But I can hear some things, like lawnmowers and balloons popping and thunder." Maybe it was my imagination, or maybe it was my sensitivity to what my son was feeling, but I got the distinct impression that my three-year-old boy was wistful. Maybe he felt that if he could hear, his mother and father would be happier with him.

In a flash of revelation, I felt that it would be wrong for Nick to get a cochlear implant. What if he grew up and thought, "My parents didn't love me just like I was, so they tried to fix me to make me more acceptable to them?"

That was certainly not the way we felt. We just wanted to be sure he had every available option, including the option to hear and speak. But I couldn't help feeling Nick would not want us to choose for him. He was happy and comfortable being exactly who he was... so we should be, too. And there we had it, our final decision: we did not get Nick a cochlear implant.

Looking back, after all of the soul-searching and the experiences we went through, we have come to several conclusions:

1) Families are all different. Every deaf child is different. Therefore, different decisions can all be valid. The question should not be, "Should deaf children have cochlear implants?" The question is actually, "Should this deaf child and family decide to have a cochlear implant?"

2) Parents have the right to make the decision for their child, even if the decision is different from the decision you would have made.

3) All of us need to accept each other's right to our own decisions and try to understand the feelings behind the decisions, whether it be for a cochlear implant, communication style, or educational placement.

4) We have a responsibility as parents to find out all that we can, and carefully consider the decisions we make. This is the first time I have written about my feelings surrounding our cochlear implant decision. Every time I write something about Nick's deafness or our decisions regarding him, I feel another release from the grieving process that hearing parents of Deaf children experience. It is especially satisfying to share these feelings with other parents of deaf children, for as we share our experiences, we heal together.

Charlotte Wilhite is a registered nurse, a part-time interpreter and has had several photographs published in *Memory Maker's Magazine*. She lives with her husband, Max, and their nine-year-old son, Nick, in Ft. Worth, Texas. Nick lost his hearing after contracting meningitis at age 10 months.

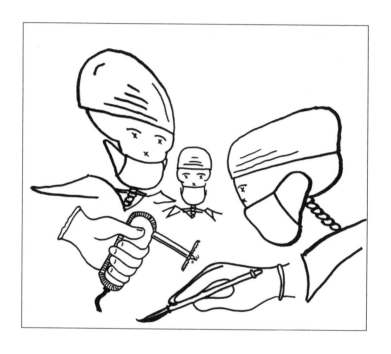

*Illustrated by Wendell E. Goff

CHOOSING DESTINY

By Marianne Decher

O Young One,
Whose name I don't even know
You are DEAF, Beautiful Deaf
The world is in your Hands

Yet pushing it aside you grasp
For impersonal hardware
That reeks of empty hopes:
"Now you will hear. Now you will speak".

Causing
Obstacles,
Creating
Havoc,
Liberty
Eroded,
Avenues
Restricted

Identity
Mutated,
Possibilities
Lessened,
Apparatus
Never
Terminable

Icy cold steel drill
Hungrily clawing at bone and flesh,
Chiseling and chipping away

At a body too young to know
What it means to
Hurl oneself over a cliff
With great faith
And no parachute.
Could it be that what you seek
Is already in your heart,
In The People who embrace your
Having been born perfectly, completely
As you were meant to be?

Let not the wire from your head
Become a strangling noose on your identity,
A tug-of-war rope between
Two worlds which can dance together,
Yet never truly marry.

The time has come
You have chosen your destiny.

Anesthetized, behind closed doors.
Surgical masks covering
Mechanized medical assembly lines.
Echoing above the scream of
Bone devouring metal probe
Is the mantra:
"Resistance is not necessary.
You are being assimilated."

Marianne Decher is an Oregon resident and a recent ITP
(Interpreter Training Program) graduate from ASLIS in Seattle. She
is the editor of another book, *Our Stories: The Soul of Sign Language
Interpreting*, also published by AGO Gifts and Publications. When
asked why she wrote "Choosing Destiny", Marianne shared the
following:

"I was a volunteer for several Deaf Programs in several schools. One of the older, elementary students caught my eye because of their expressive and fluent signing, and because of the fact that the child was so clearly Deaf! I found out that that the student's family never learned to sign and that in the next few days the child would be receiving a cochlear implant by choice. It tore my heart out. I don't remember seeing the highway through my tears during the 30 minute drive to my ITP. 'Choosing Destiny' was written for the child from that experience."

People Who Inspire Us

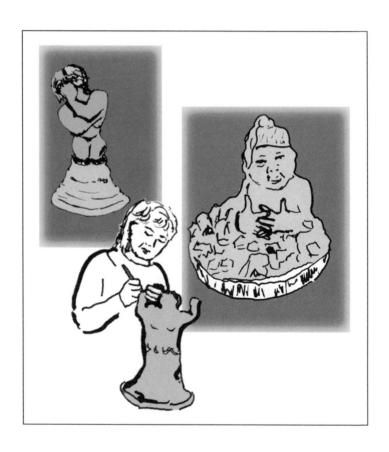

*Illustrated by Wendell E. Goff

- 100 -

Hands are for Sharing

By Michael Rosen

When a person has endured much pain and suffering, yet can still be a source of compassion and love, it is truly amazing and inspiring. Such is the case with Helene E.R. Oppenheimer.

"Rescue" has been a recurrent theme in Helene's life. Coming to America from Germany at age seven with her physically and sexually abusive father, and her developmentally disabled German-Jewish mother, Helene was eventually rescued by her grandmother and declared a ward of the California courts. She was then placed in many temporary foster homes. Throughout these difficult times, Helene would temporarily escape into the world she sketched and colored.

At age 14, Helene was kidnapped and tortured, and eventually left abandoned in a parking lot. Her perpetrators would never be caught. Unfortunately, no one was able to rescue young Helene from this excruciating experience, so she had to find her own way of dealing with the pain. She turned to drawing as a form of healing.

Helene returned to Germany to complete high school and matriculate at the University of Heidelberg. When she returned to California, she rescued her sister and two younger brothers from the same abusive household that she had endured as a child, taking her siblings into her own home. After earning her California teaching credentials, Helene taught high school German and English.

After her siblings grew up and moved out, Helene bought ten acres of the Redwood Forest in northern California. She specifically chose this location in an effort to save many beautiful trees from logging. She built her dream home there and eventually adopted several unwanted cats, providing them with a loving home. Each summer, Helene traveled the world and led student peace tours. By 1989, Helene had finally put her painful past behind her.

Then on November 3, 1990, there was another cruel twist of fate. Two cars rear-ended a vehicle in which Helene was a passenger, catapulting her into life with a permanent disability. She suffered a very serious back injury. No longer able to teach and in severe pain, Helene reached out to an old friend, her creative spirit.

As Helene explained, "Art and creativity helped me endure my painful childhood. I have had much practice turning difficult times into positive experiences. Making the best of hard times has been my main challenge in life. Like many other survivors, I have been guided by a creative spirit."

Helene added, "The accident devastated me because all I ever wanted was to be a teacher. People knew me as a good teacher and that was my whole identity. I had worked very hard to earn this reputation. With six herniated discs and chronic, acute pain, I was forced into sudden retirement. In my devastation and desperation, I turned to clay."

During her long, slow recuperation, Helene learned what it was like to have an "invisible disability." One cannot see the back pain she and many others like her endure everyday. Interestingly, this "invisible disability" wound up drawing Helene towards the Deaf community. Helene realized that many Deaf people are isolated and misunderstood, as deafness is also something you cannot see.

Not surprisingly, Helene came to identify very closely with the Deaf world. She began to sculpt Deaf, African-American women signing American Sign Language

(ASL). Through them, she was able to recapture some of her dignity and self-esteem, by sculpting strong, intelligent women emanating self-worth and dignity.

Helene also relates to the African-American culture of the women she has modeled in her sculptures, through her background as a German-Jew.

"German-Jews share many historical and cultural parallels with African-Americans," she remarks. "We have more in common than we have differences."

Sometimes, a touching movement or word of encouragement can change one's path in life.

"In 1994, a Deaf friend came into my studio when I was sculpting 'Inspiration'," Helene reminisces. "It was my first ASL sculpture. I remember how he had two distinct reactions... the first was 'oh, that's lovely, a new sculpture.' But then he had an additional look of pride, smiling in sheer delight as he recognized that the sculpture was communicating in his language."

Helene recalls how her family of German-Jewish immigrants initially struggled with this new language and culture she had become fascinated with. Her Deaf friends are native-born Americans, yet they share similar trials and tribulations. With her one-of-a-kind ASL sculpture exhibit, however, Helene welcomes the Deaf and hearing to appreciate art and culture together, building a bridge between them.

Helene credits the positive reactions of the Disabled, Deaf, and African-American communities for inspiring her to create over 40 ASL sculptures. Her growing exhibit is titled "ASL in Clay: A Sculpture Documentary with African-American Deaf Women." Her sculptures address issues such as breast cancer, amputation, Judaism, gay pride, age and size oppression, sexuality, war, Deaf hospice and spirituality... all in a positive, uplifting, and beautiful manner. She has found that while her back can no longer serve, her hands can still teach and share with others. Helene's creative spirit has indeed rescued her.

Helene's most recent rescue centered on me. If she hadn't suffered the car accident and found the strength to express her passion through clay, she would still be isolated in her forest cabin and I would still be a 48 year old bachelor here in Minnesota. But fate (and a creative spirit!) decreed that we meet, even though separated by half the country. Her tragedy and pain opened my heart and my life to love and compassion. On August 9, 1997, Helene and I married. I am now a proud husband and stepfather to her eight rescued cats.

From a life of pain and isolation, Helene's creative spirit rose above and motivated her to create wonderfully inspiring sculptures. That others have been touched by her gifts is obvious in the praise she has received for her work. Helene was recently selected to represent Minnesota as a delegate at the 1999 International Art Festival for Artists with Disabilities, which was held in Los Angeles.

Helene's sculptures have won Best of Show, and People's Choice and Encouragement Awards at international competitions. She has been named 1997 Most Accessible and Active Minnesota Disabled Artist. She was also a 1998 winning entry in their juried Fine Arts Show and was a Featured Artist this year at the 1998 Minnesota State Fair, which over one million people attended.

Yes, I am amazed, but more than that, I am grateful for the spirit that kept her going until we could be together. Together, we can share the future—Helene, her amazing creative spirit, and myself.

Michael J. Rosen, a Minnesota resident, is a former American Sign Language interpreter and is presently employed as a Speech and Language therapist in the Saint Paul Public Schools. He has written articles related to sign language interpreting for the Minnesota chapter of the Registry of Interpreters for the Deaf (MRID). He also wrote an article for the RID views about the creation of the sign language used in the movie, "The Piano." Michael enjoys woodworking and is an avid NASCAR auto-racing fan.

To see Helene's sculptures online, visit her page at http://home.earthlink.net/~aslclay or send a free ASL in Clay e-card at http://www.illustrationbydesign.com/card/send6.htm.

From an Abyss of Addiction, A Deaf Adult Child Survives

By Dr. Frank James John Lala, Jr.

Becoming a victim of alcohol or drugs is a terrible fate for any individual, and a loss for society. As a Deaf adult child of an addicted family, I was born to middle class parents in Los Angeles, California. My hearing parents, Frank Sr. and Isabel, made their living as a salesman and an IBM keypunch operator. I was a healthy, hearing child; the first five years of my life was blessed with two wonderful, loving, and devoted parents. They provided everything a child would need. Looking back, the first ten years of my life seemed wonderful. Every Christmas I awoke finding our living room filled with hundreds of balloons. Presents were piled high under the tree. I recall one special Christmas morning I found an adorable German Shepherd puppy just for me!

However, at age five, I began to lose my hearing due to an antibiotic drug (Streptomycin) intended to combat a tonsillitis infection. My parents were heartbroken at the prospect of my profound deafness, and were concerned with how it would impact my life, but they continued to shower me with affection and love. I attended a number of hearing schools before finally being referred to a Deaf program.

Eventually, I was placed at the California School for the Deaf in Riverside (CSDR) around the impressionable age of nine. "Culture shock" doesn't even come close to describing the ordeal of attending CSDR as an oralist amongst a student body of Deaf children who used sign language to communicate. Initially, I was unable to communicate with them except for primitive gestures.

Shortly afterward, while I was going through this major change in my life, my parents divorced. While I was at CSDR, twice a week Dad sent packages of goodies and toys. They would be for all my classmates or for all thirty-two boys in the dormitory! Today I ponder whether dad was just spoiling me, felt bad about the divorce, or felt guilty about having to send me to a boarding school. It was probably a combination of all three.

At the end of my first year at CSDR, Dad suddenly and tragically passed away during the summer. He died of a heart attack alone on the corner of Hollywood and Vine. At the same time, Mom was in the hospital with an acute ear infection when the heartbreaking news hit. In a bizarre twist of fate, Mom wound up losing her hearing, five years after me. How ironic this seemed, because there was absolutely no deafness in our family history except for mom's twin sister Mary, who had a similar ear infection and also became deaf. Both sisters were twenty-eight, and in their prime of life. Naturally, they met this hardship with great distress. First, they lost their jobs, which almost immediately forced us into poverty. Communication with the world, including friends and family, became hopeless and doomed. Our existence diminished to a feeling of total abandonment, and our outlook became bleak, desolate and joyless.

I sadly watched Mother become an alcoholic, just like her sister Mary had. They both abused prescription drugs. Gone were the Christmas trees, the presents, or even someone to talk with on Christmas morning. At CSDR, all the boys questioned me about the goodies and toys, which were no longer coming in. I was angry with dad for placing me in such an embarrassing situation. I struggled with the grim reality that he was gone. Because I was dealing with all these horrendous hurdles and roadblocks, I changed from an outgoing, friendly person to a withdrawn and frightened young boy. Isolation consumed me, along with hostility and anger that was yet to surface. The life I once knew became a dismal shadow that seemed to be nothing more than a fantasy.

In search of love and approval, and wanting a normal life, I began to shoulder many of the responsibilities while living at home during the summer months when CSDR was closed. Those summer months away from school were extremely harsh. I collected empty soda bottles from the streets of Los Angeles, and exchanged them for cash at the markets. Potato chips, corn chips, or pretzels satisfied my hunger pains. If I was lucky, with a good day's collection of bottles, I would treat myself to a slice of pizza or a cold, plastic-wrapped sandwich from the liquor store. There were many times that I didn't eat for two days. Sometimes, I bought a package of macaroni or spaghetti, but I ate it without sauce or butter. Once, a kind man from Ralph's Supermarket noticed my plight and directed me around the back of the store, where he loaded me up with edible vegetables and fruits, which were about to be thrown away.

Once CSDR reopened in the fall, however, my environment again became normal, healthy, and placid. The teachers cared about our learning, and the counselors advised and protected us. I had friends, and the surroundings were peaceful and unobtrusive. It was a place where I could sleep undisturbed for eight hours a night, and enjoy hot meals three times a day. It was heaven — the only real home I had — and marvelously so, not infested with cockroaches and bedbugs. Angry at what substance abuse did to my life and my family, I swore that as long as I lived, I would not drink any alcohol, use drugs, or smoke. Somehow, in this terrifying and grim existence, I wanted to help others with their substance abuse. I decided that after I graduated from school, I would pursue this dream.

Life at home continued to be difficult. On one occasion, a man attempted to break into our duplex. He broke down the door and startled Mom. She screamed, and he fled the scene. Quickly, she ordered me to get a butcher knife from the kitchen. I was eleven years old at the time, being asked to fend off a wild maniac, burglar, or worse. I stood tall trying to suck up the courage needed to fight off an intruder (fortunately, he did not return). Meanwhile, I glanced over at my mother, only to see that she had passed out from booze. Crazy with fear, I stood guard most of the night, holding on to my dear cats. If they heard anything, I'd know someone was lurking around the house.

I fell asleep eventually, and the next morning I checked on mom. She was fine, and remained asleep on the couch. I sighed in relief. The whole thing was another pitiful, but typical experience that affected me adversely.

At age sixteen, while home during a holiday break, I came home to our apartment and found it destroyed. The apartment manager informed me that it was my mother's lit cigarette that had set the fire. He threw us out. Secretly, I knew that Mom was probably drunk and had passed out. She was hospitalized with burns from the accident. For three days, I walked Hollywood Boulevard, where it was safe because of the many all-night tourists, until it was time for me to catch the CSDR bus on Sunday, in downtown LA.

The aftermath is sad. I eventually attended the funerals of my entire family (mother, aunts, uncles and grandparents). They all died of substance abuse, in one form or the other. My Aunt Mary was in a coma when my mom died from an overdose of sleeping pills. One week later, Mary passed away without ever regaining consciousness, never knowing that my mother had already died. What was so strange about this is the fact that they shared everything together, even death. They are buried beside one another.

From all of these experiences, I grew up quickly. Inwardly, I did not understand the concept of how, as a Deaf adult child, I suffered from severe psychological problems. I had experienced and witnessed alcoholism and drug abuse at a very early age, but I did not understand the concept of addiction until I was eighteen. By then I had watched Mom go through four hours of agony when I refused to give her a bottle of vodka. She screamed, pleaded, and cried. She broke out with body shakes, cold sweats, binges, blackouts and other withdrawal symptoms. I had refused to give her alcohol because she was pregnant and I was concerned about her unborn child. I wanted to nourish her and the baby, and attempted to bargain with her to eat first. She was completely at my mercy, and she looked like she was dying before my eyes. I was so apprehensive that I finally surrendered. By this time she could not even hold the bottle (or open it, for that matter). She acted like a total stranger. This was not the mother I had known all my life.

Eventually, my half-brother Daniel was born with Fetal Alcohol Syndrome, and since his birth has been a ward of the State of California. I also have a half sister, four years older than Daniel, who has a learning disability as a result of Mom's alcoholism. Fortunately, as the first child, I had been spared from any health problems because Mother did not drink at the time.

From a long and weary journey of heartbreak, confusion, and despair, I survived. Death surrounded my family, and later, my friends—all from the plague of substance abuse. I knew they had all died in vain, unless I could learn something from their tribulations. Having stared death in the face as it took all of my family members by the time I was twenty-one, I refused to become a victim or a statistic of substance abuse.

As a young man in conflict, seeking to overcome many psychological problems, the healing began when I learned how to forgive. I forgave my parents for divorcing; my father for dying much too soon; and my beloved mother, Isabel, who drank her life away because she didn't know how to cope with life's substantial obstacles.

I have fared well, despite my parent's misfortunes, and my entire family's afflictions. I certainly paid a heart-rending price, but to state it simply, I made a choice and I fought back. I remained in school and continued my education. I became one of the four co-founders of a recovery program for Deaf and Hard-of-Hearing Alcohol and Drug Abusers in Southern California. I wrote my doctoral dissertation about Deaf substance abusers with my advisors on the dissertation committee, Dr. Harlan Lane and Dr. Betty G. Miller. I have authored many periodicals regarding my stance against substance abuse.

In the area of therapy, I continue to encourage and pursue the demand for more insightful and caring counselors, intake personnel, therapists and other professionals. We need public support both monetarily, and in less tangible areas such as morale. Overall commitment on the part of everyone involved in the therapeutic process is greatly needed on both the giving and receiving ends, to enable people to bring their best to the process of eliminating the impediment of alcoholism and substance addiction from the deaf community.

I've had an interesting life full of drugs, death, and alcohol. I've buried both parents and feel I come from an overload of addictive experiences that have inspired me to help others, Deaf or not. Substance abuse is a social problem that needs to be resolved through government programs, public awareness, and education. Our Deaf citizens have many problems to overcome, and it's way too easy for them to go inward and withdraw. I know, because I was there. But through strength in my conviction, I overcame any dependency on drugs or alcohol. I am helping others follow my way, the way to a healthy, normal, self-sustaining life.

Frank James John Lala, Jr. currently lives in California. He obtained his Ph.D. in Public Health and a Certification in Alcohol and Drug Abuse Counseling from UCLA, and works as a consultant and chemical dependency counselor. He is also a freelance writer for numerous publications, and has authored *Counseling the Deaf Substance Abuser.*

Through the Eyes of Deaf Navajos

The biographies of Glenn Alfred and Karen Johnson as told to Henning Irgens and Sharon Kay Wood

Deaf individuals who are born into Native American tribes often come from bi-cultural, or even multi-cultural environments, especially those who attend residential schools for the Deaf and go home during the holidays to family members who live on the reservations. In this section, there are two oral histories of a Deaf Navajo man and a Deaf Navajo/Dine female, as told to the husband and wife writing team, Henning Irgens and Sharon Kay Wood.

Glenn Joseph Alfred

Glenn Joseph Alfred is a Deaf Native American of Navajo descent, born to a family originating as horse people, and later settling as sheep farmers. His family clan on his father's side was Naakaii, or Mexican Dine, whereas his mother's clan was Hashtl'ishnii, or Mud Clan. Rooted in tradition is the recognition of the mother's clan over the father's clan.

Growing up, Glenn recalls living in a tent amid land on the Navajo Reservation, with the sheep from which they subsisted. The family included five brothers. For shelter and warmth, they had only a wood stove inside a tent. They slept around the stove at night. Women slept on the right side and the men slept on the left side. Mother was the main force in the family, as men came and went from time to time. Glenn remembers having the ability to speak the Navajo language.

Generally, the sheep belonged to women and children. Children worked outdoors, tending the sheep by horseback. Glenn's grandfather cultivated corn for subsistence. The men used horses and equipment to dig out a pond, letting water flow in from the river for animals, plants, and other needs.

By today's standards, the family was poor. However, Glenn did not think so, as they managed quite well with hand-me-downs, sewing lots of patchwork on the clothing. He was told later by members of his family that when he was born in mid-winter, a freshly slaughtered goat was used to cradle him. He slept inside the stomach cavity of the goat, thus keeping warm, in accordance with a cultural belief that he would be given a long life.

He remembers that when he was little, children went barefoot most of the time. He remarked that his feet would develop thick leathery skin, tough enough to handle the roughness of the generally barren and rocky land where sheep roamed. In cold weather, he sometimes had his feet swathed with grass and clothes wraps.

A river flowed nearby, and they had to cross it with a raft strong enough to transport a horse and wagon used for shopping at the country store. His mother, Annie Begay, would often weave rugs from the wool sheared from the sheep. She would do lots of preparatory work such as carding, spinning, and finding dyes from plants, as well as setting up a loom suspended from trees or beams set up outdoors. Her rugs would be the means of payment for wares from the country store. Children were taught to recognize and collect the diverse plants for use in dyeing and weaving.

Glenn describes his childhood as a happy one, despite many hardships. From an early age, he had the responsibility of tending the sheep, making sure they would not stray off, and keeping an eye out for locoweeds and larkspurs that could kill the livestock. Each child in his family had designated sheep or lambs of their own. Once, he remembers being so engaged with making things with his hands that the sheep he was supposed to be herding wandered off out of sight. This brought forth the wrath of his aunt who lived nearby. Some sheep would have bells tied to their necks, so that they would be easy to locate. Glenn, being Deaf, would have to roam many miles to find them. He remembers his mother took some puppies out to live with the sheep and feed them scraps of vegetables and boiled meats, so that eventually they grew up to protect the sheep from the coyotes, which always presented a threat to the herd.

Glenn's maternal grandfather was a Medicine Man, Denetchilly Begay of the Mud Hogan Clan, who had a lot of influence on the family, and managed their property (some of which Glenn inherited later). Glenn recalls walking around with his grandfather, collecting plants and storing them for later use. He saw his grandfather as a very important figure around home, as well as in the larger community of the tribe. Glenn felt that Grandfather was a very tough man, as he would bathe himself in the snow, even when he was close to ninety years old! Grandfather had also been known as a good wrestler among the men. He chopped wood for warmth in his hut, and was also handy with rope, particularly when it came to lassoing horses.

At the age of ninety-three, due to the on-set of blindness, Grandfather got lost in a windy snow storm despite the ropes he set up to help him feel his way from the hut to the outdoors area and back. He was rescued, but nearly frozen to death when they took him inside. Grandfather later developed pneumonia, which ended his life. Glenn said that grandfather's longevity was attributed to eating the same kinds of food all of his life. His grandfather on his paternal side passed away at the age of 101. Glen says that to this day, he follows the same regimen that his grandfather did.

Glenn's father, Willie Alfred, was killed in an accident when he lost control of his horse-drawn wagon on a downhill stretch of the road. This happened when Glenn was three years old. Glenn loved to hang around the horse corral. One day when he was four years old, Glenn was walking on top of a corral fence when he slipped and fell. He hit his head on the rocks below, knocking himself unconscious. He woke up two days later and realized that he had become Deaf. He still could speak a little Navajo, but had difficulty understanding members of his family. To facilitate communication, a natural system of signs was developed and utilized by his family.

For many years, Glenn stayed at home herding the sheep by riding the horse he had owned since childhood. Glenn recalled that the saddles they rode with were typically cast offs from the U.S. Army. He would make himself a valuable helper at home by getting water from the river, feeding the horses, and tending the sheep. This he did through most of his young life, until he was nearly fourteen years of age.

Glenn also shared that his mother would dig up yucca plant roots to make soap, which could at times be rough on the skin. Also, his older brother had once visited a landfill near the town of Farmington and found a World Book Encyclopedia, with pictures that Glenn (twelve years old at the time) enjoyed looking at from time to time.

Glenn briefly attended a Bureau of Indian Affairs supported local school, but could not continue as it became clear that he could not benefit from the school. It seemed that Glenn was fated for life at home. Yet by pure happenstance, some members of his family met other Navajo people who told them about a relative with a Deaf son, who was attending New Mexico School for the Deaf (NMSD), in Santa Fe. The father of the Deaf son, Jack Kellywood, noticed Glenn communicating with his mother using in gestures, during one of the gatherings that they attended.

Later, Jack's father, an employee at one of the boarding schools, informed the Bureau of Indian Affairs about Glenn. A social worker from the Bureau of Indian Affairs, who spoke Navajo, came to see him. It was decided then that Glenn would go to the school for the Deaf. The social worker picked him up just before Thanksgiving and took him to Santa Fe, where Jack had been enrolled the year before. Glenn brought with him his daily work clothes, which were the only clothes he had.

At NMSD, Glenn was exposed to a new culture of tradition and learning. He was fourteen years old at the time. He looked with wonder about the school, its many buildings and the streets outside, all of it puzzling to him. It was quite a change from having lived in a tent for many years, having never seen constructed buildings where people lived. There were Deaf girls, male peers, and Deaf teachers that he found fascinating. His sign name was given as a "G" resting against his chin.

At first, he was acquiring new signs from fellow students. He was once taught to use his middle finger for "thank you" to staff, which created a great deal of embarrassment for him. Dr. Thomas Dillon, the Deaf principal, followed up on Glenn, and decided he was at the receiving end of a prank from some of the older boys. After that experience, Glenn grew wise to future pranks.

Among other experiences, he recalled having attempted contact with Deaf girls, which resulted in strict punishment. The consequence entailed digging a foxhole, approximately four feet wide, four feet long, and four feet deep. Upon passing inspection, Glenn would be required to fill in the hole, a task that would take many hours to complete. This lesson discouraged any further romantic contact with the girls!

At school, Glenn learned artwork, carpentry, printing, and other activities, which he really enjoyed. Today, in the school's superintendent office, there hangs a watercolor painting of the earliest constructed building on the campus, which was painted by Glenn. Also, he and other students made furniture for the school, some of which are now regarded as pieces of art. Glenn recalled that when he took up printing, he was able to type fifty-four words a minute, which was a rather unusual feat. However, he did not continue in that craft, as he preferred shoe repair work. He thought shoe repair would be more realistic for life at the reservation, and so his chosen career was that of a shoemaker.

At the age of twenty, Glenn had to leave the school due to the age regulation. By then, he had learned enough basic math skills and some reading over the course of five years. It was at school that Glenn learned to drive and was the first of his brothers to get a driver's license. After he left the school, he did odd jobs around the reservation. Several years later, his wanderlust became so strong that he migrated to California. There he was employed as a construction worker, after being encouraged by hearing Navajo friends. Working in production-type jobs, such as in an aircraft factory, proved to be interesting experiences for Glenn. There he worked as an engine lathe operator at the McDonnell – Douglas industry in Inglewood, near Los Angeles. While in California he met a young hearing Navajo woman, Rosemary, who became his wife in 1963.

With his wife, Rosemary, Glenn came home and had five children, two sons and three daughters. Rosemary became a fairly good signer and was very helpful in serving as his interpreter at his shoe repair shop, which he began on the reservation. It soon became apparent that many of his customers could not pay for his repair work. Unable to collect the money for his repair work, Glenn and his family moved away from the reservation, close to the city of Farmington.

In Farmington, Glenn and Rosemary ran a shoe repair shop for several years until it became unprofitable for them to continue, again due to the customer's inability to pay. He had, in the meantime, acquired several machines for his shoe repair work, which were rather expensive. When the business taxes he was required to pay became too high, they decided to move back to his property at the reservation. There they lived off the land, as Glenn was an able farmer. They grew vegetables, which they sold at the weekly craft market. He would often be found working in the field cultivating the soil, running water for irrigation, weeding, or taking care of the harvest. At home, he would do some shoe repair work, which added some income for necessities such as feeding and clothing the family, as well as upgrading vehicle maintenance.

In time, due to the rising cost of living, Glenn learned how to repair cars. Glenn had to use his ingenuity to locate parts for the cars, which were too costly. He would go on frequent trips to junkyards, so he could salvage parts and modify them for his relatives' cars. To this day, one can always see him driving used cars that do not have electronic injection systems. He states he does not work on engines with new electronic gadgets, but that he concentrates on transmissions and other moving parts. He carries a reserve box filled with parts in the back of his vehicles, staying prepared for eventual breakdowns on the highway. Wire clothes hangers, incidentally, happen to be very handy for temporary use until getting home!

Due to Glenn's problem solving acumen, he would often be asked by diverse craftspeople to help out with details relating to cars, houses and other technical issues. As a result, Glenn acquired a widespread reputation as a skilled craftsman of sorts, especially in building modern hogans. A hogan is a dwelling that normally has eight sides (or is an octagon shape) in the traditional style constructed at the reservation during the last 150 years. Glenn would be called in to help solve occasional problems of accurately matching joints of wooden beams, and aligning them by squares and half squares to support the roof. No architectural designs would be available, so he would have to make an assessment on how to build it correctly. From there, he would provide directions using sign language or drawings, as well as demonstrating how to complete the task.

Often workdays would be very warm, so the worker's thirst would run high. The workmen would then drink iced water, which Glenn avoided. He noticed their energy span would wane, while he could continue working consistently by sipping warm water.

Glenn occasionally mentioned that during his youth, his wrestling prowess with men in competitions was quite formidable. At times, his opponents would grab one leg to twist it around, so he had to roll over several times to avoid injury. He had to think fast to outsmart his opponents. He had plenty of strength, but exerted himself so much that later in life he developed a hernia. It required surgery to prevent part of his stomach from shooting out. This condition has to be taken into consideration when heavy lifting is called for, something he no longer wants to do. One of his hearing sons followed in his footsteps and became a good wrestler, winning the state high school championship in wrestling. His son is now enrolled as a student at University of New Mexico.

Today, Glenn is a shoe repairman with a shop in the city of Farmington. He drives off the reservation in order to open shop and supplement his meager social security income as a partially disabled person. Glenn pays support for the needs of his family, including his wife (who lives with one of their daughters who has several children). Why would Glenn continue that when they are all grown up? He hopes that in return, his family will look out for him when he becomes too old or disabled.

Karen Billie Johnson

On May 6, 1972, the world welcomed Karen Billie Johnson in the Shiprock, New Mexico hospital run by primarily by the Dine Navajos on the Navajo Reservation. The Dine Navajo are the largest Native American tribe in America today. They are located in the Northeast corner of Arizona, in a small portion of Southeast Utah and a part of Northwestern New Mexico. Karen's parents are Harry Johnson and Alice B. Foster Johnson.

She was raised in the traditional six-sided hogan covered with earth with a single doorway facing the first light of the day from the East. When she was three months of age, she fell in her home. She was brought to the hospital and it was discovered later that she had become totally Deaf from the injury.

At the Bureau of Indian Affair's recommendation, Karen was sent to the New Mexico School for the Deaf at Santa Fe (NMSD), at age six in 1978. For a long time, she was homesick, as she had never been exposed to signing hands or Deaf culture. She was fortune to have Margie Propp (her spelling teacher), and Ernest Ortego (Deaf Mathematics teacher), make her feel that she was part of the group. Later, as a teenager, Karen adored Esperanza Correa Latimer, who was the first Deaf alumnus of NMSD to teach at the school after her graduation from Gallaudet College. Karen was enrolled in her social studies class, where she came to admire her firmness and sense of humor.

In 1984, Ms. Latimer, who was currently the NMSD Museum Curator, chaired the Founders' Day in memory of Lars Larson and his two Deaf wives, Isabelle "Belle" Porter and later, Cora Dunn Larson. They were honored for their pioneering sacrifices to uphold the school during it's many years of economic struggle. Karen stated that the Founder's Day Celebration gave her a new and strong awareness of her school's history, and instilled in her a desire to preserve her culture.

Charleen Brewer, the dormitory counselor at NMSD, also helped Karen adjust to her new surroundings. Karen recalled that when she first enrolled in NMSD, she had never seen electricity, a toilet flushing system, or running water. Charleen encouraged her to put her pajamas on, unlike at home where she usually had her daywear on when she went to bed.

Karen was given the name sign "K" on the shoulder. For Navajo, there is a signed word "N" from the shoulder to the midpoint of the chest using both hands symbolize the squash blossom with turquoise necklace or shawl. Some Deaf elders sign "N" from the head to side of chin. The tribe has not yet decided on the official signed word for Navajo.

Karen's maternal grandmother, Mannie Foster, herded sheep most of her life in Sheep Spring, New Mexico. She lived without electricity and used kerosene lamps for light. In Navajo culture, the women and children supervised the herds of sheep. There were no fences on the reservation where the sheep grazed, and sometimes the herds got mixed together at the water holes. But the shepherds could always tell which sheep were theirs.

Karen was given the responsibility of tending the herds by taking them out to pasture each day and bringing them home in the evening to the sheep pens. She had to keep an eye out for larkspurs, also known as locoweeds, that could kill the livestock instantly if eaten. Karen also had to keep an eye out for coyotes. The land she lived on had an interesting mixture of desert, tall mountains and deep canyons. Karen had witnessed coyotes mauling the sheep a few times and she spent a lot of time chasing them away. She also had to report to her Grandmother if any sheep were lost. The killed sheep would be picked up for food, to be prepared in the traditional way, such as lamb stew.

In the Navajo culture, women were the main providers of food and clothes for the family. They would also earn money from weaving rugs or blankets. Clothes had to be washed by hand, and water had to be hauled from a well, located a half mile away. In order to support the family, Grandmother Mannie wove rugs out of yarn, which was spun from her sheep's wool. Her weaving is known all over the world for its creativity. Karen admired her grandmother, who occupies an important place in her memory. She had the opportunity to help her Grandmother card and loom during the summer breaks from school. She learned to dye the strands in different colors, mostly green, using sage vegetation. A loom is made from two trees or tree branches cut into logs for support posts, and weaving starts from the bottom up. Karen observed her grandmother interlacing the colored threads that carry the design across the warp. She did not have any blueprint or pattern to follow. All of her handiwork was from her own designs.

Regular trips were also made to the trading post, also know as the pawn shop, to trade rugs or jewelry for food or other needs. Eventually Karen learned to appreciate the art of weaving and cooking. Her specialty is making fry bread, a skill that she learned from her mother.

Karen's family, or clan, is traced through the maternal side. There are over 75 clans. Their purpose is to regulate marriage. Marriage within a clan would not be allowed. The family once discouraged Karen for dating a hearing beau who belonged to her own clan.

Karen's parents often took her to the annual tribal fair. The fair featured a rodeo, singing and dancing ceremonies, as well as a craft sale. Following the fair, they would take her to Santa Fe for another academic year. This became the family tradition until she graduated in 1991. Travel to pow wows and other ceremonial events provided a rich experience in observing cultural programs. Now she is exploring her culture through reading and asking the elders and friends to fill her in on the missing information that she did not receive as a child.

Shortly after her high school graduation, Karen had the opportunity to learn about silversmithing at a local college in Shiprock. She learned that around the year 1900, the Navajo silversmiths began to put turquoise stones on the jewelry. She did not complete the course due to a lack of sign language interpreters. About this time, she was injured by a serious automobile accident near Red Valley. Abuse of alcohol was the cause of the accident. Following the accident, she was flown into the Albuquerque Hospital where she recuperated for a few months. A brace was clamped onto her head. For a while she had a memory lapse. After this experience, Karen strongly stated that drinking and driving do not mix!

Traditionally, various taboos and beliefs of religious origin have dominated Navajo life over the years. Over time, some have diminished in importance, while others are still observed today. Generally, it is considered an insult to point anything at another person. Karen learned it was proper to point at anything when she learned American Sign Language at NMSD. Coming home for vacations, she would use pointing for identification, which was very much frowned upon. She never knew it was a part of Navajo custom, for her parents spoke only Navajo.

One of her older brothers had learned some sign language from her, and would do some interpreting between her and her parents. He was the only one of her five brothers who was willing to learn ASL. This enabled Karen to understand that she was living in a bi-cultural environment, with different values and unwritten customs. At home she would pass a cigarette, a pencil, a knife or anything with a point held upright so it could not point at anyone. At school she was free to point.

For younger Navajos, life is different than the quiet life their grandparents knew. Although many Navajos follow the old ways as closely as they can, Karen agrees that some of them have newer rituals, like the use of herbs such as Mormon tea for indigestion. She thinks that the school and the community should work together in teaching about the Navajo and Dine traditions and customs as part of the curriculum. This would help to develop the Deaf Navajo children's pride in the native values and contribute towards creating high self-esteem and respect for family and tribal culture.

She hopes that the next generation will be able to embrace both cultures equally, by placing an emphasis on the positive aspects of both cultures.

A few years ago, Karen went on an unforgettable trip to the Colorado School for the Deaf and Blind in Colorado Springs, where she was invited to be a presenter on Navajo and Dine culture and customs as a part of Deaf Awareness week. It was an unusual experience for her to share her cultural history with young Deaf children and adults. This opportunity encouraged her to work toward the goal of promoting a better understanding of the diversity of cultures.

There is a story of the Spider Woman, Na'ashj'eii Asdzaa, who taught the Navajo how to make a loom. Even more importantly, Spider Woman taught the young Navajo how to use the loom. Karen feels that life could be richer with the knowledge of one's culture, which will inspire people to take pride in their history and background. She states: "Preservation of my culture and religion will help me to be a better role model for future Deaf children of my race."

Sharon Kay Wood was born in Lewinston, Idaho, and graduated from the Arizona School for the Deaf. She graduated from Gallaudet University with a BA in 1968, and obtained an MA in Deaf Education from New York University in 1983. Wood and Marjoriebell Holcomb co-authored the book *Deaf Women: A Parade through the Decades*, published in 1989. Wood has been a teacher in schools for the Deaf for over 25 years. She currently lives in New Mexico with her husband, Henning Irgens, and is working on another book about Deaf Women in the USA.

Henning C.F. Irgens was born in Oslo, Norway, and graduated from the Norwegian School for the Deaf. He earned a degree in Education, History and English from Gallaudet in 1957. Irgens, now retired, served the Michigan Department of Education as a Deaf Consultant. He also served as Project Director of Deaf Services at

State Technical Institute in Michigan for more than 20 years. Currently, he serves as a member of the Board of Regents of the New Mexico School for the Deaf.

The husband and wife team writes for various publications, and present at national and international conferences of the Deaf. They adopted four dogs and two cats, most of them imported from Norway.

Michael's Freedom

By Damara Paris

Over twenty years ago in a small village in India, Michael was born to hardworking parents who were poor. Born Deaf and with behavior problems, he did not go to school and was not able to communicate with anyone in his village, except for those who used a few home signs. The one person who had the most influence on him, and kept him from running wild in the streets, was his mother. Unfortunately, when Michael was 8 years old, she passed away.

His father, already overwhelmed with work and caring for his other children, did not have enough time for Michael. Soon, Michael was out on the streets, gradually moving up from mischief and pranks to stealing an odd fruit or article of clothing from shop owners. Unable to deal with the situation, the father contacted the police and gave up custody of Michael. There were no social services, no laws, and no educational systems available to help Michael. The solution was to put him in prison.

Michael had a horrible time in prison. Unable to hear or understand spoken and written communication, he was often beaten by the guards for his lack of response. In addition, he suffered abuse from the other prisoners. His survival skill was to play the clown and entertain people. Over the years, he had learned to smile through his pain.

After a few years in this system, he and several other prisoners decided to break out. They were caught in the process of running from the prison. Unfortunately, Michael did not hear the guard tell him to stop and was shot in the back.

Michael remembers waking up in the hospital and being tended to by Mother Teresa. It took a bullet, but finally he was able to get the help he needed. After his recovery, he was sent to an orphanage. At age 13, one year after he escaped from the prison, he was adopted by an American couple.

America had a lot of things to offer Michael. He was fed, clothed and had shelter-- even his own room. He could interact with other Deaf people and go to school. He flourished in many ways, from gaining weight to obtaining social skills, and eventually a job. By the time he left school at age 19, he was able to express himself enough in sign language to interact socially with other Deaf individuals, although he had a limited ability to communicate through written means.

Like any young man, the one thing that symbolized freedom and adulthood was a car. This was Michael's dream, since he had first laid eyes on an automobile. Every cent that he could save from doing odd jobs, was put away for the purpose of obtaining a car.

Michael's difficulty was in passing the written test to obtain his driver's license. His command of the English language was minimal and his ability to understand and communicate in sign language was barely adequate for a DMV test. He demonstrated that he understood laws and the rules of the road, but could not seem to convey this to the DMV test administrators, not even through oral examinations with sign language interpreters.

This did not stop his determination to pass. Many of us saw him go through the driver's manual every day, asking questions, underlining sentences, making diagrams. His single-minded pursuit of what he considered the ultimate freedom was both touching and heart-rending to watch.

One day, when he was 22, he came to my work place. A huge grin on his face, he took me by the hand and led me outside. Parked by the curb was a gray 1990 Nissan Sentra. "Mine," he signed. Seeing the puzzled look on my face, he pulled out his wallet and showed me a driver's license in his name. After 11 failed tests, Michael explained, he had finally passed his written test two weeks earlier. Confidence buoyed, he "study, study, study!" until the day before the exam, when he borrowed a friend's car and took his performance test—and passed. That morning, he had taken the bus from his apartment a final time, gone to a dealership and wrote out a check for the entire amount of the cost of the Sentra. This represented three years of strident saving while he pursued his dream.

I was honored to be asked to ride in his car down to the nearest McDonald's for a lunch treat. A Big Mac was never more enjoyable for me than in that moment.

Damara Goff Paris lives in Oregon with her husband and 16 month old daughter, Sekoia Dawn Paris. Paris is currently employed by Oregon Public Utility Commission as the manager of three telecommunications assistance programs. She is also the owner of AGO Gifts and Publications and writes freelance for other publications, including *DeafNation Newspaper*. Paris is currently working on two projects, *Deaf Women of the Pacific Northwest* and *Rotic Weekends*, a novel.

World War II in Norway

By Henning Irgens

I was born Deaf to a hearing family and grew up learning to understand and speak a spoken language. My ability to communicate was limited, until I enrolled at a state school for the Deaf in Oslo, Norway.

It was during World War II. Norway was invaded and occupied by the German Forces from April 9, 1940 through May 22, 1945. Long before 1940, we had seen newspapers full of stories of German military maneuvers occupying various parts of Europe. When I was a child, we could see pictures and read text of Hitler's activities, such as the "Brownshirt Bullies" pressing upon minorities in Germany. We read about Hitler's trusted men, such as the highly effective PR man, Goebbels; the activities of the German Luftwaffe's hero Herman Goering; Ambassador Von Papen's secret diplomatic overtures; Von Ribbentropp's foreign alliance movements that lead to the takeover of Austria, Sudetenland (a part of Czechoslovakia) and other smaller countries.

I was ten years old in August of 1939, when I traveled throughout Northern Germany with my father. We visited our ancestral town of Itzehoe, the place where our ancestors were born before they relocated to Norway and began our branch of the family tree.

While there, I vividly remember the Brownshirts rushing by in cars and trucks. This gave me a strong feeling of fear, and a sense of insecurity, which I later labelled as "war mood." On the way back through Germany, while traveling by train, I saw troop movements traveling eastward near Kiel. I noticed a civilian, an older man, following my father and I until we reached the border of Denmark. Later, I came to understand that it was the custom that foreign travelers in Germany would have older German males following their movements. It was only a few weeks after this episode that I understood the reason for the massive troop movements on the trains going east. It was during the "pretend" quarrel over Danzig in Poland, which started World War II in September of 1939.

I also remember reading about the umbrella-carrying Englishman, Chamberlain, who was in Munich signing an accord of "détente" with Hitler to refrain from future aggression. Norway also participated in the accord, making efforts to preserve its status as a neutral country. During this time, Oslo newspapers had features about German spies in Norway who had been arrested for activities such as gathering information about maps and defense installations. One German name I could remember very well as a child was "Ratenfels." To me, no matter how horrible a spy he was, I felt his name was pretty because it was so easily pronounced.

Life remained uneventful until the night of April 9, 1940. I was at the state school for the Deaf located several miles outside of Oslo, in the forested, uphill country. The older boys, including myself, were sleeping in a large room that contained about 25 to 30 beds. During the night, some of us were awakened by large airplanes flying low, so low that we thought they barely missed the Norwegian anti-aircraft cannons as they passed over the tall spruce trees swaying in the wind. A hard of hearing friend named Hans, who later became a champion Olympic skier many times over, came to me and together we sneaked out of the room and got up into the loft, where we placed chairs to stand on while peering out into the opened skylight. And what a sight it was!

We saw a brief air dogfight, but mostly we witnessed dots of smoke in the weak moonlight where cannons peppered the sky in an effort to down German airplanes, which we could identify by their double black and white crosses. We saw parachute soldiers sailing down from high, only to disappear into the woods. That night, we all developed stomach cramps caused by the fear and reality of war. We heard the reverberations of powerful cannons and the roar of junker style planes. Some of the Deaf kids crawled under the bed in fear. The women house parents, with whom we could not communicate well, were nowhere to be seen but later showed up to explain the situation with the help of some of our hard of hearing peers.

Later, during a day lost to sleep and worry, my older sister (Sis) had telephoned a message that I was to prepare to come home. She lived and worked in Oslo and had taken the streetcar to pick me up at the school. Together, we traveled to the center of the city of Oslo.

It was there that I witnessed a sight that I have never forgotten. When we got out of the underground streetcar station, we started walking down a big street. There were German soldiers lined up along the curbside training their machine guns upon civilians who walked down with their suitcases and backpacks. Sis and I walked with our hearts in our throats to the railway station, where we boarded a train traveling some three hours to our hometown south along the coast of Oslofjord. At home, our parents, who had seen nothing of the gruesome display of war reality that I had just seen, welcomed us. Due to my lack of ability to communicate, I was not able to describe the scene I had left hours ago.

Nearly two months passed before we saw the first German Occupation Force moving about our town. At the time, I was happy to be home, and felt secure in the absence of war mentality. Newspapers were controlled and told nothing of the war movements in Norway. My family would listen to the radio (which was later confiscated by the Germans and members of the Nazi party), but could not tell me much. The neighbor boys took pains to explain what was happening. I was able to tell them in limited fashion what I had seen on the night of April 9th.

Life went on rather tranquilly as those of us who were young pursued soccer playing. My mind became occupied with dribbling the football. It was not until fall, when we were called back to the state school for the Deaf, that I became increasingly aware of the true extent of the war.

That fall, we had a male substitute teacher. Our regular teacher, who had gone to the United States for a visit, was unable to get back into Norway. At that time, sign language was forbidden at the school. However, braving the potential wrath of the school officials, the substitute teacher combined both sign language and speech in his story telling and took us far away from the realities of the impending war. He told us stories of his childhood, of living in Africa with his missionary parents, of facing the dangers of reptilian invasions as well as dangerous animals such as lions and leopards. Those tales took us away from the fear of war for six wonderful months.

When the regular teacher arrived, we were once again entertained, this time by her tales of traveling by train from New York to San Francisco. She mapped out the interesting landscape she covered, managing to teach us to study the map of America. Upon hearing tales of cowboys and Indians, we developed a penchant for adventure in America. She used the oral approach, but proved to be very efficient in relaying information to us. Our class consisted of the same classmates with the same teacher, who became sort of a mother confidante, teaching us in all subjects over an eight-year period.

Due to the increasing scarcity of food and clothes, we were on strict rationing. As the five-year period of German occupation evolved, our food supply dwindled, so we had to cultivate more vegetables in the field, as well as in galvanized buckets filled with soil and organic wastes. The potato became the king of survival. We had hot potato porridge for breakfast, potato soup for lunch and fried potato "steaks" over and over again, day after day, with an occasional supply of fish. Bread was scarce because much of the food in Norway was taken to support our "Masters" fighting out in the eastern and western fronts. Clothes had to be mended and recycled into hand-me-downs. Sugar did not exist but we had saccharine, a substitute sweetener in the form of tiny pills found in pocket sized wooden boxes, similar to snuff boxes. We carried these around to use for adding to drinks or even coffee, which was made of scorched beans or grains. During the war, dentists had fewer customers, as we had almost no cavities due to the diet we were living on.

I remember having dry skin, which was paper-thin, and one could see the tiny veins through. It often happened that the other boys and I would go skiing and brush into the branches of spruce trees, getting scratches on our hands and faces, and leaving open wounds that would take many weeks to completely heal.

Occasionally we would get our hands on boxes of sardines, which we would hide in our knickers. There was a limited supply of such luxury items, and we hid before eating them, sharing only with our best friends. Since the school required a complete blackout of lights in buildings, the rooms were completely dark, and we would have to feel our way around to the bathroom. I remember opening a sardine box under the cover of my blanket and eating the entire box, which was drenched in olive oil. The next day, those of us who had eaten the sardines could see a slight transformation of our dry skin to a normal hue, and a complete healing of our scratches. But that would not continue for long.

Once in a while, we would observe the women personnel in the dorm, as well as in the kitchen, and noticed that they were well fed, rotund and healthy. This raised suspicion among us brighter boys that they had helped themselves to the food that was designated for the Deaf children at the school. At least once a week, when we had terrible hunger pangs, some of us would take turns going on secret missions downstairs to the basement where the kitchen and food storage were located. We would put on our knickers and move stealthily along the wall of the stairs, not touching the banister, then wait for the night watchman to come out of the locked kitchen door. We would move behind the door as he walked past us up the stairs, and just as the door would close, one of us would move in quickly, letting the door close slowly to give off the normal sound of shutting. After waiting a few seconds, we would sneak inside the kitchen area and stock sandwiches into our pant knickers through the knees, and then move cautiously back to our bedroom hall, sharing with those who could keep their mouths shut about our stealing. We did that for a time until we found our fingers painfully caught by big rat traps placed inside the steel containers holding the pre-prepared sandwiches. By that time, disease was found rampant among the kids living in the cold damp stone buildings. I had a slight touch of illness and, to my joy, was sent home before Christmas, along with many other students.

Those of us who were sent home missed school for half a year. My mother decided I was not to be allowed to loaf around and took me by ear to the dining room table where I was forced to read. To her horror, she discovered I that I had not learned the fundamentals of reading.

Although I could grasp the content, I was sorely lacking in the implicatory aspect of what I read, and I had difficulty reading "between the lines." That was when I came to a better understanding of her language and more capable of understanding spoken Norwegian than any of the other foreign languages that I was to learn years later.

Thus, I was learning more at home than at school, which proved that home was more conducive to learning, especially since my parents had thousands of books in our home library that filled four walls. I could not help but delve into the various sets of encyclopedias. I soon earned a reputation for being a "walking encyclopedia."

Returning to school was sort of a pain, but I enjoyed the comradeship, and growing up with both girls and boys sharpened my sense of what I was and what preferences I was to develop. I completed school by confirmation as the custom was, for all education was designed to help us understand the bible as a fundamental guiding factor for future living. At the age of fourteen, I found myself at home. I spent some time at my younger sister's farm. She and her husband had met at the university, but it was closed during the war as required by the Occupation Forces. The Occupation Forces feared that the university was a breeding ground for more intelligent resistance to Nazism. My sister and her husband decided to buy a farm and conduct agronomic work, where I found myself working as a farmhand.

It was a peaceful existence and the food produced from the animals was good. We had cows, pigs, and chicken, as well as various vegetables and grains such as wheat and oats. Working as a farmhand, I developed a rugged constitution. I did stable cleaning, tilled the fields by horse drawn plow, cut big birch trees, herded and milked cows, hayed and completed harvesting of soil products (such as grains and potatoes, sugar beets and other important foods to be stored in underground caverns for winter sustenance). It was hard work for a fourteen-year-old boy who became a man early. Also, the years I spent on the farm made me a voracious reader of most of the classics that I had missed at the state school for the Deaf.

Because of that positive experience, I had gradually built up an "inner language" from reading that enabled me to speechread very well, by anticipating the context of words spoken by non-deaf people. On the weekends, I spent time away from the farm with my parents, who lived in town. During the winter when there was not much work expected of me, I stayed at home.

Then the German High Command in our town demanded occupation of our house, which was cradled higher up the mountains with a gorgeous view of the fjord. This was possibly to insure that their officers would not be harmed living with us. Thus, we had six German officers living with us, occupying three of our bedrooms and reserving one of the bathrooms for their sole use.

We would talk with some of the homesick officers, who would engage in conversations with my parents because they were fluent in German. This created a friendship with some of them that continued by letter exchange long after the war was over. These officers proved to be well educated and some of them were real scholars. It was then that I developed a high respect for their knowledge, although they were "hedging" under Nazism as proselytized heavily by members of the Nazi party in Norway as well as the Gestapo, which was the German security police. Generally members of the German Army would show great respect for Norwegian individuals with an educational background, so my parents were left alone.

After two months, however, the High Command gave an order for us, my parents and I, to evacuate our home to provide a living habitat for more officers. They found an apartment downtown that had been vacated by our town's newspaper editor, whose family had fled secretly to Sweden, a neutral country. They were wanted for questioning related to suspected anti-political activities against Nazis. We lived in that apartment for one year until the war was over.

Because I had no Deaf friends living in my hometown, I would seek the company of hearing friends, who often gathered at a local canteen to sip pop. They were high schoolers, and talked a lot about school issues. My association with them whetted my curiosity for learning at their level, which I quickly found was similar to my own abilities. Sometimes I would show ignorance about difficult topics, much to their amusement. I noticed that the less learned teens were the ones who laughed at my ignorance because it made them feel that they were a notch above me, which they did not fail to point out. There were areas where I had inadequate knowledge, such as expressing myself in acceptable spoken Norwegian. Nevertheless, I formed deeper relationships with those who had greater maturity. It was with these friends that I was able to associate. As I became more aware of the cultural patterns of the hearing community, I was able to mingle quite comfortably among my peers. In fact, I adopted a kind of bi-cultural posture because of the two worlds that I was living in. Occasionally, I would meet older Deaf adults, with whom I could communicate using signs, which felt more natural and unrestrained than the communication I had with my hearing peers.

While living in town, I found myself getting into mischief with a few hearing boys my age. Once, we found that a German had parked his military BMW motorcycle by the wayside, and two of us decided to "borrow" it! We would take turns running the powerful motorcycle up and down the snow-clad road, skidding around fast turns. My friend went up the road while I stood waiting for his return. Soon I had a pistol stuck up my back, held by a German soldier! As soon as my friend came down about halfway, I waved my arm to warn him, which he saw in the distance, and he jumped off the motorcycle, disappearing in the plowed snow heap by the side of the road. As the soldier ran to catch my friend, I saw my chance to disappear into the snow, and I dove into the soft heap, burrowing into it. I could hear pistol reports shortly after I went into hiding, but I stayed mouse-still in the snow long after, until I felt safe. When I could hear (through vibrations) the motorcycle rumble away, I rose up and walked a circuitous route back home, shaking but not telling my parents about the escapade.

During the week I would bicycle up to the farm, which was located in another county. For traveling from home to my sister's farm, I would have to have passport clearance from the German High Command. I would go to the farm when we needed supplies, to get food such as smoked bacon, ham and eggs, as well as meat cuts, all of which I carried in my backpack.

Once, I was approaching a curve around a knoll not far from home when I found myself stopped by the German Security Police. There was a line of people, walkers and bikers, carrying bags and backpacks, who were being searched for contraband items such as food, war important items, illegal weapons, or parts for radios or other electronics. Up on the knoll was a machine gun nest, and another one was down by the side of the road. People were nervously opening up their bags for confiscation. I was stopped and was about to open my backpack when the inspector was distracted by some commotion in the crowd. I saw a chance to close up my bag and put it on my back, as if having completed inspection. I waved to two soldiers standing up front with rifles at the ready. Casually, I began riding my bicycle, pedaling easily, then gradually speeding down the road. Soon, I heard and felt the vibrations of the deep rumble of the military BMW motorcycle being started up and when I dared to glance back, I saw two soldiers holding up machine guns, one on the cycle and the other in the sidecar!

Fast and furiously, I pedaled down the hill and had to go around another curve shielded by tall spruce hedges when I saw a chance to go uphill, a hill that I normally would walk my bike up. But fear lent me powers unknown and I raced fast uphill to another curve and around a jutting residence before taking a different route to my parents' house.

I did not tell my parents about the incident, but being hot and wet, I bathed and changed into fresh clothing, then rested a while before sauntering down to a neighbor's house where my best friend lived. He told me that he had heard a machine gun spraying nearby not long ago, so I assumed that it had been intended for me!

During the winter doldrums, there was not much socializing allowed due to the dangers inherent at night. Some evenings I had to dress like a man and accompany my sisters to parties so that the Germans would not accost them—as the Germans had a reputation for bothering single women on the road. Other times I participated in a weekly chess club. This was our only diversion other than reading. One time, I had stayed late because a strong opponent played well against me. As I left the club after the game was finished, there was total darkness on the street. I was stopped by a machine gun on my belly and then a light flashed into my face. A German soldier was in front speaking, so I said what I had learned as part of my survival lessons, "Ich bin taub" pointing to my ears, and of course holding my hands above my head and then showing my passport identification. I was let go after he screamed loudly "Auf!" which I saw and heard faintly. I still had to walk along the wall side of the street, as it was dark. Soon a cloud parted, allowing the moon to shine so I could see more clearly with the snow reflecting the light.

Passing an alley, I saw a German standing with an open long coat wrapped around a struggling woman or girl. I saw at once that he was attempting to rape a Norwegian. I started making several hard snowballs, fortified myself with them, then approached the German, bombarding him with the hard snowballs so he had to let the female go—who then proceeded to run out of the alley. The female shouted a "thank you" to me as she left, or at least that is what I guessed she had said.

I ran up the street and ducked into a recessed door of a town building and saw the German in the long military coat walking by. I was shocked to see it was one of the cultured officers whom I had met at our home prior to the time that we had been driving out of it the year before! From that time on, I became wary of "educated and cultured" people. I understood they were all minds, with little or no soul. Today, I see the proponents of pure oralism in the same way, supporting an ideal, yet exhibiting a total lack of human caring for the needs of Deaf people. It was an enemy who taught me that concept—at only fifteen years of age.

The war years taught me many things, mainly through observation. Prior to the war I saw people who were upright Christian turn into members of the Nazi party. These individuals held onto the idealism of social equality through moral mind power, keeping the race pure as propagandized by Goebbel's machinery. They were the ones who actively reported on any perceived anti-Nazi behaviors of Norwegians. They were the ones that would help round up hostages in the event of the sabotage of bridges, ships, or war machinery. They would also drive big trucks to pick up people wearing anti-Nazi colors such as those on the Norwegian flag— red, blue and white. I recall having lost one red cap, which I wore to show my patriotism, and as a result, I spent a few hours in a very crowded jail.

Before the war, I used to play with boys who came from alcoholic homes, or homes where their fathers were out at sea sailing around the world on freighters, or on whaling ships from our hometown. These boys were rough and uncouth and were looked down upon, but they were still friendly with me. I could see beneath their exteriors that they were good, and I showed no fear of them as my other neighborhood friends did. The neighbor boys had older brothers who were very courageous, showing strong patriotism by working underground, doing sabotage work, and blowing up railway bridges used for German military war material. These men formed a resistance that often suffered a loss of life by execution or torture. Along with men of all other classes, they lived in the mountains and forests, surviving by their wits. Sometimes good folks would venture up and provide the boys with food, as my sister and her husband did. They had to be very careful so as not to be caught by spies or the Germans. Since I was one of the few who had a transit passport from county to county, I once had a mission as a carrier to bring a radio part from a family acquaintance to another person near my home. I was not to know their names as I could reveal them if I was caught or tortured. Fortunately, I was not caught, but there had been many times when I was routinely stopped to have my bag or passport searched.

The war ended in May of 1945, and there was much celebration, as well as "witch hunting" of Nazis, fraternizers, and women who had consorted with them. We saw them being paraded on the streets, some having had their heads shaved and stripped of the belongings that they had acquired from patriots during the war. Our home was found in a terrible state. The furniture was damaged from drunkenness and lascivious living by German soldiers and German women, or "gray mice" as we called them. We had to fumigate the whole house, replace the tapestry, wall texture and repaint the walls and doors, repair some of our antique furniture, reupholster sofas and chairs, and touch up paintings that had been sprayed by liquor or other things. It took us several weeks to do the necessary repairs before we could move back into our home.

In the house I found helmets, gas masks, belts, and leather holsters for holding weapons, which the former occupants had left. The underground civilian Norwegian soldiers, with the help of English and American soldiers, rounded up the German military and had them shipped back to Germany by midsummer.

It took five years for Norway to get back on its feet and produce the food and clothing needed for general living. When I entered Gallaudet College in 1952, I worked at the Washington Post Weekly at night to earn extra money. I bought food packages and some clothes to send to my parents, who were grateful for the gifts I sent overseas. Thus ended the indelible experiences I had as a Deaf person during the war years in Norway.

Henning graciously submitted his story involving his post-war experiences in the next chapter. Please turn the page to find out more about his life after the war.

Post-War Experiences
of Henning Irgens

By Henning F. Irgens

World War II ended in April of 1945, after German Forces surrendered unconditionally to the Allies in Europe. By the first week of May, the German officers who had occupied our home had to vacate our house in the hills and were taken to a prison camp for deportation to Germany. They had used our home as a means of protecting themselves against the Allied Forces, who would not bomb the homes of Norwegians. We found our house in great disarray, probably because the officers had conducted drunken orgies upon learning the news of Hitler's death. Whether they celebrated the end of the war or the prospect of returning to their homeland is not known. German "WACS", uniformed women, had also lived in our house. We used to call them "the gray mice" for the color of the outfits that they wore.

Fumigation for lice and other insects, due to lack of cleaning during the last days of the war, was necessary. It took a few weeks before my family could move back into our house. Summer was very strange for us, for there was a new feeling of freedom after five years of oppressive German occupation. Patriotism ran high when our King, who had fled Norway upon the German "Blitz Krieg" occupation in April of 1940, came back to his castle in Oslo.

During that summer, the Norwegian underground "civilian" army continued hunting for people who had fraternized and collaborated with the German Forces during the war. Norwegian Nazi members were rounded up, and their property and materials that were acquired by unlawful methods were confiscated. They faced either the criminal courts, or trials of treason against Norway, after which they were imprisoned.

Some Norwegian women who had consorted with the German soldiers were hunted out, had their hair shaved, and were paraded on the street through a throng of angry people who hurled insults, rotten vegetables, and spit. Weeping and red faced, with their clothes torn, they were cursed. After that, they were no longer seen, for with shaven heads they did not dare go out in the open, except perhaps at night. Some of them found refuge with relatives up on isolated farms, until they grew longer hair. Some of them had babies from consorting with the Germans, and some of them were allowed to join the soldiers they had lived with and move back to Germany with them. Some came back years later, with new names and children, to live under more tolerant conditions, concealing their identities. Life was not easy for them.

Some Norwegians had profited during the war by contract work or business supply distribution designed for the German Forces. With the wealth they gained, they had purchased the expensive homes and farms. However, after the war, they were forced by the new Norwegian Government to relinquish all of the property that had been bought with the income from working for the Germans. Some of the worst of the group fled to South America under false names, so they could not be hunted out. Some of the more clever individuals had hidden their fortunes in Swiss Banks, and were able to start new businesses elsewhere in Europe and in South American nations, like many other Germans with war crimes on their records. A Deaf friend of mine had a father who had grown immensely wealthy and he fled to Argentina, where he was never seen again.

That was a summer of strange events. We found out that some people who we had been missing during the war turned up either alive or dead. Some had survived German concentration camps, where they were found alive under stacked up piles of dead prisoners. They had blinked their eyes to catch the attention of the Allied Forces soldiers, and were saved in the nick of time. Others missing were found in mass graves in the woods with their hands tied behind their backs, executed. I knew two of them, for they had been boyfriends of my two older sisters before the war. They had worked secretly in the Norwegian underground army, and had been in hiding because some of their ranks had been unlucky enough to be caught and tortured by the Germans.

For that reason, many members of the secret army used code names for identification so that their fellow workers would recognize them. I remember recognizing a young man, who was a fiancé of a girlfriend of one of my sisters, at a street car stop in the capital city of Norway. I called out to him using his real name, Finn. He wouldn't acknowledge me and I was puzzled, seeing how he so persistently avoided me. He kept shifting his eyes, looking around to see if any Nazis or German secret police were present.

I felt hurt by his behavior, for I used to be on good relations with him and his family. I told my state school for the Deaf teacher about that experience, and bless her for her wisdom, she explained about the underground forces, which required the use of false names. I was made to understand that Finn had been lucky to get away without being killed. This experience made me aware of the need for greater sensitivity during the war. I saw him again after the war, wearing a military uniform and smiling. These young men were heroes of the war because they survived under a veil of secrecy and they often did not have enough warm clothes or food (farmers would be executed for collaborating with people working against the Germans). It was a time when everyone had to take every precaution not to give out names or other pertinent information.

By the end of summer, there was still a shortage of food and clothes, so care had to be employed in preserving food for the winter. Food rationing by stamps was still in use for a couple of years after the war. At that time I traveled to a western city in Norway for vocational training. I was sixteen years old, and I had completed 8th grade at the state school for the Deaf in 1944. At the vocational school, I met old school mates and other young Deaf men from various schools in Norway. There I was consigned to taking up the tailoring trade, which I disliked very much, but had to accept, as there was no other choice.

Meanwhile, because no Deaf girls lived in the city, we took to dating hearing girls, which offered us some diversity. The school did have a dormitory, but there was not enough room for some of us, so we lived in rental rooms with families in the city. Dating a hearing girl who attended a local high school whetted my interest in the subjects she was studying.

That was the beginning of my interest in pursuing academic training, for I found myself helping the girl with understanding her English textbook instructions along with other subjects she was studying. The girl's mother wondered why I did not attend high school, which I explained was not accessible to Deaf students. I was encouraged to attend high school, so I approached the headmaster of the vocational school with my request. Fortunately he was one of those rare teachers of the Deaf who said "Why not?" I was given private instruction in

English on a trial basis with a woman teacher, who reported to him that I would make a good student despite my hearing loss.

Consequently, I left the vocational school to go back home and apply for admission into the local public high school. I was denied entry, as the superintendent had known me since my childhood, and he felt that I would be disruptive to learning in the classroom because of his perception that I would not be able to follow spoken instruction. However, a mother-in-law of my sister, who was a schoolteacher, and a friend of the Superintendent at another city, persuaded my parents to consider her school. I was admitted on a trial basis, where I did reasonably well even though I could not understand any of the lecturers who presented in the high school gymnasium.

Due to the fact that my 8th grade level education from the state school for the Deaf was weak, I had to have private tutoring two hours a week to strengthen my ability to tackle foreign languages, advanced math, and writing. Those sessions helped me to clear most of the hurdles that were presented in regular public high school, and I completed the program in five years instead of the usual six years. During those years, I had to take daily train rides back and forth from home to the city school. Sometimes I would miss the train, so I would bicycle many miles in order to report to class. A couple of times during the winter, I would be forced to take a short cut, skiing a lot of terrain, which took me about two and a half hours when I missed the train for school.

At the end of high school I had to take both written and oral exams to obtain a high school certificate to qualify for university study. All of the exams were universal for all Norwegian high schools, in written format, but there would be random oral exams in some of the subjects. I was able to clear all the written exams but was very nervous about the oral exams, where two independent lecturers from other cities appointed by the Norwegian Department of Education who would be conducting questions.

In my case, I had to take three oral exams, one in English, one in German, and one in Natural Science. Fortunately, I had spent three weeks one summer at a student camp in England where I had practiced with English speaking college students, many of whom came from Scotland, Wales, and Ireland, with English as a second language. This helped me speechread them and converse somewhat meaningfully with them. In addition, my English teacher had Deaf siblings and knew how to sign. This helped me considerably with reading about English history and becoming familiar with English literary writers, which I had to demonstrate knowledge of when responding to verbal questions from the examiners. As a result of these two factors, I obtained the top grade on the English oral exam.

In German, I did well, having read a lot of German literature, but the oral exam consisted more of conversational skill in responding to issues where I had to couch properly spoken phrases to demonstrate my knowledge of German grammar. I passed Natural Science with ease, thanks to my collection and knowledge of the 900 different plant species put into a herbarium, complete with written Latin names and descriptions of each plant. The questions generally would require identification of some plants and the proper Latin names for them.

As to my speech ability, I did have weekly speech tutoring in all of the languages I had to learn. Lipreading, or speechreading for that matter, was quite tough but a bit of imagination and helpful memory for speech articulation helped me a bit.

Following completion of all my exams I was awarded a certificate by my high school as directed by the Norwegian Department of Education. This qualified me for university study. I was at first offered a stipend to take up studies for the legal profession, which I felt was beyond my ability (especially since interpreting services did not exist back in 1940's). I felt that I had to decline, but asked if I could enroll at the Teachers' College. That was denied because the oral medium employed at the time dictated that all teachers working with Deaf children must be hearing. This left me in a great quandary as to what I could do, so I worked in a factory making windows and doors for one year. During that time I learned about Gallaudet College in a Swedish newsmagazine for the Deaf, so I wrote to Gallaudet for information. I applied, with the goal of becoming a university librarian. Having saved up some money from my factory work, and with financing from my parents, I was able to travel by cruise ship from Oslo to New York.

I carried two suitcases and one carry-on bag, plus one thousand dollars in my pocket when I entered the famed Ellis Island and was waved through on a student visa. Taking a taxi from that place to Penn Station was an experience, as I had to resort to writing and sign gestures. Passing through the streets of New York was a bit of a shock, especially with the sight of police officers carrying holstered revolvers directing traffic. Did New York still have gangsters? I had seen many American movies at home. Searching for a train from Penn Station to Washington, DC took time due to communication through writing. It seemed that the people at the station were somewhat familiar with Deaf passengers, as they were able to give me intelligible messages. Traveling in the Pullman (as opposed to European) compartment was revealing. I took to studying passengers on the train, observing their behavior. I wore a double-breasted suit with a hat, which made me feel somewhat uncomfortable. I remember seeing a young red-haired girl sitting in a bench two rows ahead, who chewed gum and appeared somewhat bratty, acting bold and unconcerned during the train ride. Many years later, I recognized her as the well-known movie actress, Shirley MacLaine!

The Union Station in Washington, D.C. was equally impressive because of its largeness, and the massive stone work all around that represented the capital of America.

I hailed a taxi to take me to Gallaudet College. It was a very hot day and I was decked out in a suit and hat, carrying two heavy suitcases and a shoulder bag. Seeing students milling about on the greens talking in sign language so fast and natural caused me to stare at them. I asked them where I could find the office and they pointed out the main entrance. Soon, I was directed to the house of the College President to a third floor apartment unit, where five other foreign Deaf students lived. There I met my future roommate, a young Englishman from Loughborough. We became fast friends and had much fun observing both the American language and sign language that varied from different states represented at the college.

It was a culture shock for me to meet several American Deaf students who were excellent signers, expressing themselves quite naturally, easily conveying ideas and general concepts. Among some of them, I noticed they did not have full command of their native American language, nevertheless they were quite articulate with idea associations. Picking up sign language came naturally to me, so I did not have to take classes in that area as some did.

Attending classes was interesting, although they were not conducted at the European level, as I had expected. The class I enjoyed the most was English, for the teacher was excellent, with much skill in signing, as well as in mouthing in proper English. That helped me to learn colloquialisms quickly, which enabled me to express myself more fluently with my fellow students.

On weekends I worked at the Washington Post newspaper, inserting colored flyers before distribution. That allowed me to earn some extra money for my personal needs. Once I went to the Washington Post to collect my weekly check and I found people waiting in line. There I saw an interesting young woman, who stared at me for a long time, and made me feel somewhat uncomfortable. Later I found out she was a newspaper photographer and reporter named Jacqueline Bouvier, who would soon marry the man who would become President Kennedy.

I met several Deaf students in the dining room where we happily conversed, most of which revolved around questions about my own country, background, and culture. As time went on during the first year, I became close to a Deaf lady, Betty Louise Lydick from Pennsylvania, who was in her last year of college. She was very bright and well read, and became my tutor in initiating me into the overall and complex American culture, which I soon came to appreciate. She got a teaching position in New Jersey, where I visited her once a month as my funds permitted. Two years later, we married. I still had to complete four years of college, as Gallaudet did not allow acceleration to courses to complete a degree in less time.

My summer work consisted of using handyman skills, such as painting, carpentry and roofing details. During my college years I was fortunate enough to get scholarship support from a Rotary Club in New Jersey to finance my complete education.

Majoring in Education of the Deaf became my choice over Library Science. The requirements for the Education field in the United States were not as restrictive as in European universities, so I took advantage of the opportunity. Betty had agreed to my request that she study the Norwegian language so that we both could go to Norway to teach in state schools for the Deaf. This we did. Upon completion of my training at Gallaudet College, Betty and I took jobs teaching at the North Dakota School for the Deaf. One year later, we traveled by boat with our firstborn son Jarl, to Oslo, where we spent the whole summer with my parents and the rest of my family. Inquiry with the Norwegian Department of Education indicated strongly that Deaf teachers would not be accepted to teach in academic courses due to observance of the speech requirement. Four years later, we again applied for teaching positions in Norway. There were forces among hearing teachers at my old state school for the Deaf who opposed the idea of Deaf teachers even though my former teacher was secretly supportive of me. We returned to the United States, as we could no longer set our hopes on Norway, the beautiful country of my childhood.

Thus, we decided once for all to forget our dream of working in Norway, and instead devoted our lives to working in the U.S. Over the years we taught at a state school for the Deaf. The pay was not good enough to allow us to consider graduate school, so when an opportunity presented itself, I applied for a Federal Fellowship in Deaf Education. I used the most reasonable argument as to why I, as a Deaf person, should apply for it as it was seemingly geared to hearing people. Among 500 or so applicants, I was one of two Deaf persons selected for National Leadership Training in the Area of the Deaf at California

State University at Northridge, where I also obtained a Master's Degree in School Administration and Rehabilitation in 1964.

There were ten of us studying under a very stimulating learning program, utilizing full time interpreting services for the two Deaf participants. We were so grateful for the interpreter services, as it afforded us the opportunity to associate and collaborate with the eight hearing professionals in our classes. It provided us with many insights that broke down the subtle barriers of the "it's us or them" mentality. That experience made us more sensitive to hearing people, opening up friendships that lasted for many years.

After completion of our studies, we applied for jobs. We sent many applications, complete with resumes, nationwide. The fact that I was Deaf seemed to turn off many potential employers. Eventually, upon encouragement of a Deaf Chief of the Department of Communicative Disorders in the U.S. Department of Vocational Rehabilitation, I applied for a position as a consultant with a vocational technical program with rehabilitative services in Michigan. During those years I was not able to find any suitable professional jobs in other states. So I worked in Michigan in the same capacity for twenty years, until I retired in 1984. The climate back then was not favorable towards Deaf professionals. Our school had not received the kind of financial support necessary to expand, due to the political forces in that state, so I was glad to leave in hopes of finding a new career.

In the meantime my wife, who had received training in computer work at my school, had obtained a very good position with the Federal Government U.S. Defense Department. She worked as a computer systems analyst with an option to retire in five years. Therefore, I decided not to apply for jobs outside of our state, and I looked for jobs in our neighborhood. I soon found that I was too old and too Deaf to "qualify" for a full time teaching job where the educational philosophy was basically oral, and the practice was to use only hearing teachers. However, having been certified to teach in nearly every subject from middle school to high school, I was able to work part-time as a substitute in the regular schools. This worked out as I could give verbal directions to students for classroom assignments, and help them individually from desk to desk with whatever problems they had. It was quite an interesting experience. I saw individual differences among several minority groups, some being disadvantaged by poor basic education or limited home environments. Income from this job soon created tax problems for me, so I was advised by a tax consultant to leave that job unless my employer was willing to let me work full-time.

A few years later my wife, who had commuted to work twenty-nine miles one way each day, had a auto accident as a result of black ice on the road, and she died instantly. Only a week before, we had purchased a motor home and planned to spend our retirement traveling in it. Her sudden departure left me very confused. I could not grieve much, for the shock was too great. It took me a month to deal with my grief, after which I decided to rig up the motor home and tow a "dinghy" jeep for a long trip out west. I spent some time at my daughter, Heidi's, in California, staying with her for two months, until I decided to drive back home. There I sold the motor home, for it proved to be too big for me, and I purchased a smaller one, which I kept for about ten years to use for sporadic travels across the U.S.

Loneliness drove me to visit places, including Gallaudet University, where I met a new friend, Sharon, through the introduction of Marjorie (Mabs) Stakely Holcomb. She later became my wife. Mabs was our "best woman" at our wedding ceremony that took place on a yacht that cruised around the San Francisco Bay area.

Both Sharon and I have been working on the development of material for her book on Deaf women. We opted to move away from the fast life in the east for a more quiet location out west. That turned out to be Farmington, New Mexico, where Sharon's mother and brother live. Four years ago, we designed an adobe style home that was custom built atop a mesa, with a view of three states in the Four Corners area. I hired four carpenters and worked with them in the construction of our home, which was completed in six months. The house was built with three garages, one of which would have our motor home parked inside. We lived in that motor home while working on interior carpentry and floor work, which took time until we moved into the living quarters.

Currently we are both active in community affairs in the state of New Mexico. Sharon taught in a public school working with two Deaf children of Native American descent. Soon one child transferred to the state school for the Deaf, and the other to a program under the Bureau of Indian Affairs. Since then, Sharon has taught ASL at a local college in Farmington, which she still does on a part-time basis.

I was appointed by the state's Governor and approved by legislation to serve as a member of the New Mexico Board of Regents with New Mexico School for the Deaf. Coincidentally, a Deaf student I had studied with at graduate school in California many years ago had been a principal of NMSD for nearly a lifetime (unfortunately, he had retired and passed away by the time I came on the scene to serve as a regent for the school).

As for future goals, Sharon and I hope to do some more traveling. We also intend to pursue additional studies for our own enlightenment. Life is a tremendous growing experience, and we intend to keep on growing.

Henning C.F. Irgens was born in Oslo, Norway, and graduated from the Norwegian School for the Deaf. He earned a degree in Education, History and English from Gallaudet in 1957. Irgens, who is now retired, served the Michigan Department of Education as a Deaf Consultant. He also served as Project Director of Deaf Services at State Technical Institute in Michigan for more than 20 years. Currently, he serves as a member of the Board of Regents of the New Mexico School for the Deaf. He currently lives in New Mexico, with his wife, Sharon Kay Wood, and their four dogs and two cats, most of which were imported from Norway. Both Irgens and Wood write for various publications, and present at international and national conferences of the Deaf.

FRIEDA AND ME

By Ira J. Rothenberg

A woman named Frieda Zimmerspitz Wurmfeld died on Saturday, October 14, 1995 (one day after Friday the 13th!) from a massive heart attack at the age of 85. What is it about her that warrants a place in this story? Probably nothing more than the fact Frieda was our family friend for many years—59 years altogether. The last time I saw her was on Thanksgiving of 1994. I thought I would see her again on the following Thanksgiving, but she passed away before then. After receiving the news of her death, I was stunned, and could not believe that she was gone. She was a link to my family history. With her passing, I feel that a part of my past is gone, too.

Frieda, the last of seven children, was born on July 22, 1910, in Slovakia, to Salamon Pinkus and Cecilia Schindel Zimmerspitz. *(To help the readers, who may not aware, Czechoslovakia no longer exists. Slovakia achieved its independence in 1992 from the mutual split with the Czech Republic. Bratislava is now the capital of Slovakia and Prague continues as the government seat of the Czech Republic).*

Frieda was a good friend of my deaf grandparents, Julius and Henrietta Benedikt Gross, in Bratislava. For a while, Frieda's former husband, Ludovik (Lou) Wurmfeld, went to the Jewish school for the Deaf with my grandmother in Vienna, Austria, which was about 40 miles from Bratislava. Frieda went to another Jewish school for the Deaf in Budapest, Hungary as the Viennese school was already full. This explains why my grandparents and Frieda didn't really become friends until adulthood. Bratislava was also where my hearing aunt, Renée Gross Hartman, and my deaf mother, Hertha Gross Rothenberg

Myers were born, respectively. In spite of their deafness, they all were multi-lingual. In addition to spoken languages (German, Hungarian, Slovak and some Hebrew), they also used a mixture of German and Hungarian sign languages. Frieda knew all of my grandmother's immediate family. Furthermore, to demonstrate Frieda's connection to my family, she told me that my great-grandfather, Eugene Benedikt (who was also deaf) conducted a ceremony to formally witness Lou and Frieda's engagement.

Everything ended sadly when the Nazis took over Czechoslovakia and made life miserable for many Jewish people. The Nazis forced them to relocate to a ghetto. They wanted to contain them to make it easier to deport them. Of course, most Jews didn't fully grasp the situation until much later. Often, they were ordered to squeeze into apartments already occupied by other Jewish families. When Frieda and Lou received a summons from the Nazis to relocate, Frieda rushed over to my grandparent's, as she preferred to live with them. They became co-tenants with my mother's household by necessity and by choice. They had two daughters, however, the younger one did not survive infancy. The surviving daughter's name is Cecilia (or Cece for short).

My grandparents felt it was safer for my aunt and mother to live in a Christian home in order to protect the identity of our religion and culture. My grandfather knew a Deaf, Christian couple (oddly, they had a Jewish name of Weiss) who had a farm outside the city of Bratislava. He moved my aunt and mother there. Although they had shared the apartment with my grandparents, Frieda, Lou and Cece decided to hide out elsewhere for awhile. According to Frieda, my grandfather complained about the hardships of having to hide out (he was 22 years older than my grandmother). He decided to go back to the apartment with my grandmother in tow. It was a fateful decision that he made, because upon their arrival, they were arrested and deported to the concentration camps (I don't know where my grandfather was sent, but I was told that my grandmother was last seen standing in line outside of the gas chambers in Auschwitz). When Frieda found out about what had happened to my grandparents, her first thoughts were of my aunt and mother. Frieda's attempts to hide them under the cover of two different Christian households (one at a farm, and another at a Deaf shoemaker's shop) fizzled due to Aunt Renée's lack of cooperation. Whenever Aunt Renée made things difficult, Frieda was sent for with the hopes that she would succeed at convincing her to cooperate. Aunt Renée was a willful child (and truthfully, she had a mouth to match). She was given to talking back, which didn't help the situation.

Because Aunt Renée was stubborn, she decided to search for my grandparents. My mother had to follow her because she was the younger sibling and had no choice. They found themselves in Sered, which was a kind of ghetto or transition area, and they became trapped there. To make a long story short, they rode in cattle rail cars to Bergen-Belsen, a concentration camp, near Hannover, Germany. Eventually, Frieda and her family were also deported to a camp. She later told me she felt that someone had betrayed them to the Nazis. My mother and my aunt didn't see Frieda and her family again for a long time.

After nine months of imprisonment, the British soldiers liberated my mother and aunt in the spring of 1945. It is ironic to note that Anne Frank had died at the same camp only six weeks before. My mother and Aunt Renée went to Sweden first to recover, and then to reside. For three years, they lived in a series of orphanages in Bergsjö, Torekull and Billesholm. My mother went to a school for the deaf in Stockholm called Manilaskolan, and Aunt Renée remained in Billesholm. My mother's teacher at Manilaskolan had a special fondness for her. He was the nationally renowned Nils Bergström. Mr. Bergström was well known among the educational and older deaf communities in Sweden. Mr. Bergström tried in vain to adopt my mother, but she successfully resisted his plans, for she had always wanted to move to the USA. Had she been adopted, she might had never left Sweden, wouldn't have married my father in the USA, would not have given birth to me, and I would not be here to tell this story.

Also, the Wurmfelds returned to Bratislava after the liberation. Lou set up his own tailor shop with a few employees. From Sweden, Aunt Renée decided to send a letter to my grandparents. She did not know that they had already perished in the camps. A neighbor found the letter and gave it to Frieda and the Wurmfelds, who were then living in my grandparents' old apartment. She read the letter but she was puzzled by the fact my aunt had used the Bratislava address as the return address on the envelope. She took it to the Hebrew Immigration Assistance Society (HIAS) and asked them if they could track down the source. HIAS investigated further and told Frieda what they found, that my aunt's letter had come from Sweden. Frieda responded to Aunt Renée. They wrote to each other from time to time from that point on.

Meanwhile, again through HIAS, our American relatives discovered that my aunt and mother were still alive, and living in Sweden. They contacted my mother and aunt. From there, Aunt Renée asked our cousin, Goldie Pollak Kohn of New York City to send a package of donated goods to Frieda and her family because she wanted to express her gratitude toward the Wurmfelds. Being a deeply religious woman, Cousin Goldie felt it was a *mitzvah* (a commandment or duty) to carry out Aunt Renée's request and help other Jews who were experiencing hardship. She did mail out the package. Frieda appreciated the gesture. After three years of living in Sweden, my aunt and mother immigrated to the United States on a propeller-led airplane in 1948. They landed in New York City.

Esther (Frieda's oldest sister, who had hidden out for three years during the Holocaust and then settled in Paris after the war) found that Frieda and her family were alive. How Esther discovered Frieda is another story, which still amazes me, because it happened through a favor by a small group of soldiers whose nationality remains unknown. After their reunion, Esther became the impetus for the Wurmfelds to move to Paris. They had another and more pressing reason for wanting to leave Bratislava: the encroachment of the Communist Party. Upon arrival in Paris, they surrendered their Czechoslovak passports and remained there for three years.

Meanwhile, Cousin Goldie shipped out a few more packages to Frieda and her family. Frieda wrote back, saying that she was grateful for her kindness, but felt she didn't need any more assistance. However, she asked Cousin Goldie for a favor, to see if she could find Frieda's uncle, who was a baker in the States. Cousin Goldie placed a notice in the bakers' union newsletter with Frieda's uncle's name and her own telephone number. In such a big city, Frieda's uncle was amazed and intrigued to see his name in the notice. He called her up and asked for the reason behind the notice. Cousin Goldie explained that his niece, Frieda, was trying to track him down. From there, Frieda succeeded in making contact with her uncle. Eventually, the Wurmfelds immigrated to the USA. My mother said during that period although they were physically apart from Frieda and her family, their lives were still interconnected, particularly through Cousin Goldie's generous efforts.

After they all had settled down at Uncle Zimmerspitz's home in New Jersey, it was time to enroll Cece in a school. Frieda and Cece went to the Lexington School for the Deaf, in New York City with their cousin Ruth, who acted as their translator. After having met Mrs. Seitock, the admission coordinator, and completing the necessary enrollment papers, Frieda asked if my mother was a student there. Mrs. Seitock's curiosity was piqued, and Frieda explained her association with my mother's family in Europe. So, Mrs. Seitock picked up the telephone and was talking into it, but never said yes or no directly to Frieda's query. Most Deaf people can read other people's facial expressions for visual cues or responses, Mrs. Seitock remained straight-faced, which perplexed Frieda. But then, Mrs. Seitock's eyes went to the door as if she heard something behind it. Frieda followed Mrs. Seitock's gaze, and saw the door opening slowly, then to be flung wide open. There stood my mother! She was so surprised. She signed to Frieda, "You're here!"

Although they knew they were still alive after the Holocaust, my mother never dreamed that the Wurmfelds would come to the United States. That occurred in 1952. It had taken eight years and many miles across the Atlantic Ocean to find each other again. Upon their reunion, Mrs. Seitock and Cousin Ruth were so overcome with emotion that they burst into tears. From that moment on, my mother's and the Wurmfelds' lives were tied together.

Frieda had seen my mother dating young men that were drawn to her attractive looks and personality. My mother used to go out with Morton Steinberg (who now lives in Los Angeles). Morton's mother, Helen, was really

- 164 -

fond of my mother, and hoped that her son would someday wed her. When my mother started seeing my father, Herbert, Helen tried to prevent them from continuing to date by telling Frieda that my father was a gambler (which in those days carried a stigma). Because I knew Helen, and because she had always treated me graciously, I don't want to give the impression that Helen did that out of meanness. Rather, she thought she could influence the situation in Morton's favor. In any case, it was true that my father enjoyed playing cards and betting at the horse track. Frieda believed Helen's story. And being a true *yenta* (Yiddish for busybody), Frieda tried to discourage any thoughts of marriage. Fortunately for my mother, she had the ability to make her own decisions and chose my father anyway. Frieda, Lou, and Cece were at my parents' wedding. My parents lived in the same apartment building as the Wurmfelds (one story below theirs) in Brooklyn, New York, for four years. Incidentally, whether or not you call this coincidence, I was born on Morton Steinberg's birthday.

When my parents returned to their new apartment after their honeymoon, Frieda immediately went up to my mother and insisted that she meet Frieda's guest from England. Having just arrived home, my mother did not feel up to it. True to form, Frieda wouldn't take no for an answer. Eventually, my mother gave in and went up to Frieda's apartment to meet the guest, named Eileen. It was a decisive encounter, for Eileen and my mother became great friends ever since.

Eileen and her friend, Gloria, wanted to visit Paris from their home in England and asked another friend (who immigrated to England from Hungary) for a recommendation on someone who would provide hospitality in Paris. That friend, who knew Frieda during her school days, asked Frieda if she would be willing to accommodate the two young English ladies. Possessing a generous nature, Frieda agreed to put them up. This was how Eileen got to meet Frieda, Lou and Cece. When the Wurmfelds moved to America, Frieda wrote Eileen and told her that she was welcome to visit them again in the "States". Eileen later accepted this offer.

Eileen eventually met a deaf American man, Fred Katz, and married him. Later on, with their sons, they became my family's neighbors. The Katz family are Orthodox Jews and my family members are Reform Jews. The difference is the degree of observance of religious laws, traditions and customs. Orthodox Jews really observe these practices to the "T," such as keeping the Sabbath and a kosher kitchen. On the other hand, the Reform Jews are more assimilated than the Orthodox Jews, thus the observance is looser. Yet, that never stopped the Katz from being friends with my family. They never judged us. They've invited my mother as well as the Wurmfelds to all of their four sons' weddings and always included us in their Passover *Seders* (feast). They were also guests of my youngest sister, Sara's, wedding. This is an honorable testimony of endearing friendship between Eileen and my mother, whose beginnings were brought on by Frieda.

Eileen had a piano that belonged to a friend of hers. She was supposed to be holding it for him until he was back on his feet and had a place to put the piano. Unfortunately, he was killed in an auto accident. The piano stood in the Katz' apartment for many years. Frieda, who was not the type to keep her opinions to herself, often asked Eileen why the piano was in the apartment, taking up space, and "when are you going to get rid of the piano?" Eileen possessed a very sweet nature and would simply tolerate Frieda's unsolicited comments. Ironically, the day Eileen finally found a way to give away the piano, was the day that she learned of Frieda's death.

My mother has a story about Frieda that is either humorous or not, depending on how you look at it. One day, coming home from Brighton Beach (which is located next to the better-known Coney Island Beach in Brooklyn), Frieda was suffering from a bad case of windburn. My mother, who was then in her late teens, suggested a remedy, which Frieda tried. She liberally applied cooking oil and sprinkled an abundant amount of salt on Frieda's body. Frieda thought it would alleviate the windburn, but she soon realized it was like a searing fire on top of it. To this day, my mother still thinks it was funny. I asked her why she did such a naughty thing. She retorted that it was Frieda's own fault for believing in everything that my mother suggested!

One of the times that we were invited to Frieda's for the Passover Seder, I discovered that Frieda knew and could say all the Hebrew words for the 10 plagues. It was amazing for me to see the extent of her Jewish education, because in many ways she seemed more American than Jewish.

She was a skilled cardplayer, and often played cards with my mother and other folks, mostly at the Brooklyn Association of the Deaf (now renamed as Brooklyn Society of the Deaf) clubhouse. She was a chain smoker, and we could visualize her at a poker table with a cigarette dangling from her mouth. In spite of this seemingly sedentary pastime, she could be really spry and mobile. She also went out to many social functions. She traveled throughout Europe and the Middle East a few times. She liked to spend money on outings, as she felt that it was important to enjoy life.

I am not trying to portray her as a saint. She did many things that infuriated a lot of people. She could be a pest, and aggravating, obnoxious, dogmatic, uncouth, easily misunderstood, inquisitive, opinionated, and bold. Despite all this, she was never dull. Although people often felt frustrated, no one in our community could hate her. They loved her in their own ways, and were deeply touched when they learned of her death. You could say her faults and antics made her memorable!

Because Frieda had a burial plot in New York, her body was brought to the East Coast. It was at the Katz' home that Cece had the *shiva* (a traditional Jewish sitting only when a death in the family occurs) so that a central place was available to accept visitors, especially long-time friends in New York. To me, it was like a full cycle of coming home. It began for Eileen as Frieda's guest in Paris and New York. And then the roles were reversed, where it was Eileen's home in Brooklyn that Frieda fittingly became a final memory, as manifested in the *shiva*.

In some ways, I felt that Frieda was a surrogate grandmother to me, somehow taking the place of my real grandparents, who did not survive the Holocaust. In addition, she had known five generations of my family (she knew my grandmother's parents and their siblings; I'm in the fourth; and my nephew, Justin, is presently the fifth). Frieda had seen my mother go through her pregnancy with me as well as with my younger sisters. She had been around for our births. She had watched us grow up. She came to our birthday parties, holiday dinners, my Bar Mitzvah, and my father and stepfather's funerals. When we wept, she wept with us. We even went to the same spot at Brighton Beach, where many deaf people congregate during the summers.

Although she moved to Las Vegas, Nevada in 1994 (I moved to California in September 1983), I still feel that our connection is based in Brooklyn, New York, which was our hometown for many years. During the time I grew up, the deaf community in New York City was comprised of mostly first-generation Americans. Many of them carried on the values and ethics of the Old World (Europe). The values and ethics that they believed in were education, responsibility, good and honest work, family, and helping others in need. They felt that these qualities are essential to "life, liberty and the pursuit of happiness" in America. In many ways I was exposed to, and absorbed these same values and ethics. These are not only part of my upbringing, but a part of my psyche and my memories of Brooklyn. I feel that Frieda represented the continuity of the work ethic and the successes of the immigrants and first-generation Americans. Above all, I feel that she represented where I came from.

Ira Rothenberg currently resides in California and attends the UCLA Extension program to work on a certificate in graphic design and computer graphics. He has published several stories, including "Roze Gebaar: Love Speaks All Languages" in *Wilde Oaks* (a publication of DeFrank Gay and Lesbian Community Center in San Jose, California) as well as two poems in *World of Poetry*, a publication of college students.

Marjoriebell Stakley Holcomb

By Sharon Kay Wood and Henning Irgens

"If you can look back on your life without regrets, you have one of life's precious gifts."
— *Marjoriebell Stakley Holcomb.*

Marjoriebell "Mabs" Stakley was born on July 8, 1924, to a Deaf couple, Hazel Ethel Pike and Samuel David Stakley, in Akron, Ohio. The name she inherited from her grandmother, Carrie Bell Stakley. "Bell" was added to her first name, Marjorie.

Akron is known as the rubber capital of the world. Nationally known companies like B.F.Goodrich, Goodyear, Firestone, and Mohawk run their businesses by mass-producing tires and other rubber products for the world in Akron. At one point, this city attracted a large number of Deaf people, who soon found jobs in Rubber City, which eventually created a strong community rooted in Deaf culture. It became even larger during both World Wars, when hearing workers were drafted into military service, leaving openings for Deaf people to fill. It was a blessing to many who were able to buy their own homes, and also purchase cars. Naturally, a rich Deaf culture blossomed, with a variety of Deaf talent. There were crafts people, "Barrack lawyers," creative culinary experts (particularly among Deaf women), and the occasional theatrical shows staged by local Deaf actors, which often focused on sophisticated themes.

Mabs' parents, Hazel and Sam Stakley, often provided vaudeville programs for entertainment to raise funds for World War Two. Sam was also a magician. The husband and wife act traveled throughout Ohio, visiting

Deaf clubs or other organized social events. They designed and painted their own stage props and other effects to enhance their shows, which included Yankee Doodle songs. Many of the shows utilized a combination of dancing and sign language. Hazel and Sam earned praise from the Deaf community for their talent and generosity.

It was into this environment that Mabs was born and raised. Having that kind of cultural exposure reinforced a lifestyle similar to a tribal or village environment, where friends of her family were "aunts" and "uncles." Thus Mabs, like any other Deaf child of Deaf parents, grew up with fewer disadvantages than Deaf children who had non-signing, hearing parents. Hers was a natural progression of assimilated values, tradition, morals, and general education, which provided her with a head start early in life, instilling in her a strong sense of self-awareness as to who and what she was. Mabs was ready to learn earlier than usual, a fact that predicted her future success as an educated woman.

Her mother recalls trying to teach Mabs how to fingerspell her long first name, but she could only handle M-a-r-j, so it was "MJ" fingerspelled for years, with the "M" in the air descending to "J" near the chest. Two years later, her sister Lois May was born, and she was the only hearing person in the family. They were inseparable during their early childhood years. Among the values her parents had impressed upon their daughters was to always be ladylike and friendly to everybody, and to show sensitivity to others.

Mabs did not start school until she was six years of age, which was deemed appropriate by educators at that time. Normally Deaf children were not admitted for formal education until after seven years of age. She was enrolled at the Ohio School for the Deaf, (OSD) in

Columbus, Ohio. This was a city that later became known as a center of learning for scientific and technological advances. The school for the Deaf was founded in 1829, 43 years before the 1873 opening of the Ohio Agricultural and Mechanical College. That college was provided by a Land Grant Act in 1862. It was later renamed Ohio State University. Many teachers at the Ohio School for the Deaf earned their teaching credentials at that University.

The Ohio School campus occupied a central setting in the city of Columbus, surrounded by the State Capitol building, theaters, museums, art galleries and the Carnegie Public library, all within walking distance. This permitted teachers to take their classes on educational trips around the town. One of Mabs' teachers at OSD was a movie buff, and would fill her students in on the new "talkie" movies that they had seen over the weekend.

During her first year at school, Mabs spent more time in the Infirmary than in the classroom. She had been exposed to all of the standard childhood diseases. She remembers Miss Sharp, who was her first-year teacher. Miss Sharp spent hours teaching her speech and speech-reading. She had a basket filled with balls, tops, shoes, dolls, fish, and other items. Her students were expected to correctly pronounce the name of each object she pulled out of the basket. Sometimes she let them pick the items for their speech-reading lesson.

Soon Mabs moved up to the second grade in the middle of the school year, excelling in arithmetic. The second grade teacher, Miss McDonald, made her feel welcomed in her class. The girls accepted her slowly, but the boys were angry.

Miss Larmi, her seventh grade teacher of Finnish descent, was one of the teachers who graduated from nearby Ohio State University. Her teaching methods were very advanced for her time. Her techniques were so excellent, that they have become widely used in today's curriculum. The school principal visited her class daily, just to see her work. Mabs and her classmates had Miss Larmi twice, in 1937 and 1939. Marriage later took her away from the school.

In high school, Mabs rotated classes so that she had the opportunity to enjoy various types of teaching and personalities. She was exposed to the best and the worst of the teaching staff during the school years of 1939-43.

Ohio School for the Deaf offered several sports programs that provided excitement during the school year. When Central States School for the Deaf had a Basketball Tournament at the Knights of Columbus Hall during her sophomore year, Mabs and her longtime class mate, Irene Hodock, were trained to be cheerleaders for the tournament.

School life generally was easy, except for the shortage of money and clothes for many students. Girl Scout uniforms were not available for everyone, but the girls took turns wearing the two uniforms that were available. Weekends were spent with movie lovers rushing to the movie houses in the city. Since money was sometimes scarce, they often visited museums and other public institutions nearby. Mabs remembers with fondness that she and her girlfriend loved to do "window shopping," and they would walk into the most exclusive stores and imagine that they were purchasing the goods.

Mabs' observation was that students at OSD were more fortunate than other schools for the Deaf in regard to methods of discipline. Rules were strict during those days, such as no "necking" and only talking across dining tables was permissible between the boys and girls. In the auditorium, the boys were seated on one side, and the girls on other. On occasion, they amused themselves by giving novice teachers a difficult time.

Going home was limited to Christmas and summer. Mabs looked forward to spending time with her younger sister, Lois May. Her sister would show her around the house, explaining any changes made during Mabs' absence.

Lois May often complained that she had to run when called by voice to do things, yet when she wanted something from her Deaf family members, she had to walk over to get their attention. One morning, when Mabs yelled for her sister, she did not respond. Lois May had decided to ignore her. Mabs kept on yelling louder and louder. Finally, Lois May could not stand the racket and she came over to tell Mabs to "shut up," as it was embarrassing to have neighbors several blocks away hear her Deaf voice. Mabs has been silent since that day.

Once Mabs caught her mother telling a friend that Lois May had been pestering her about where babies came from and that Mabs never had never asked her about that, which puzzled her mother. Mabs smilingly remarked she had got all the information from the older girls at her school.

In her recollection of the most influential of relatives, Mabs names her Deaf Aunt Eulalia Stakley Burdick. She was an employee at the Goodyear Tire and Rubber Company, and she provided a positive female role model. Aunt Eulalla was a great comfort to Mabs when she was small, and she read and explained information to her from printed comic strips. She often clipped the strips and mailed them to Mabs at school during the academic school year. Aunt Eulalla also taught her to crochet, and to appreciate the finer things in life,

Mabs' class of 1943 consisted of five girls and three boys. They had started their freshman year with almost 50 students. Many students had left to work in the profitable war plants during World War II. Several came back for visits, especially to show off their pay slips, which were many times over the pay of their schoolteachers'.

The greatest event of Mabs' life was when her schooling came to an end on May 8, 1943. Due to the rationing of foods and materials during the war, the school year was shortened by one month, so classes were held on Saturdays to make up for the lost days. Graduation time was very touching as the students wept over leaving each other after so many years of living and schooling together. Mabs recalls:

"We had grown close, like sisters and brothers. The shared confidences, the secret fun, and the mischief brought us to tears upon our departure. We senior girls wept openly when we knew we were parting for good. The boys were somewhat confused and embarrassed. Our Senior Class motto was very fitting: Life is now our School."

The Ohio School for the Deaf had been accredited for its quality of teachers and the curriculum it offered, which enabled Mabs to enroll at Gallaudet College in Washington, D.C. It was there that she met her future husband, Roy Kay Holcomb, a classmate from Texas.

Mabs did well at Gallaudet, and during her senior year, was elected Head Senior. Mabs had once wished to work in the male dominated field of chemistry, but at the thought of handling acids that might ruin her clothes, she chose an education major. During their senior year, Mabs and Roy wrote letters of application to various schools inquiring about coaching work for Roy and teaching positions for Mabs. A contract was offered from South Dakota School for the Deaf that allowed them free room and board, which was an exciting offer for them. They looked for Sioux Falls on the map, and found the location of their future residence. They had to ask the superintendent for permission to take the time to get married before taking their positions. Their wedding took place in Akron, Ohio on September 6, 1947.

Later, along with Roy, Mabs taught in other schools for the Deaf in the country, such as South Dakota, Tennessee, and Indiana. During the summer months, Roy and Mabs drove all over the United States visiting schools for the Deaf. Mabs took pictures of Roy standing by the school signs at the entrances. They enjoyed the inexpensive hobby of travel, and in time, Roy started writing a series focusing on the history of various schools for the Deaf in *The Silent Worker* magazine, which was published by the National Association of the Deaf. Roy later wrote for *The Deaf American.*

On March 10, 1953, at the age of 24, Mabs' beloved hearing sister, Lois May, passed away in a hospital in Ohio after a lingering illness from a severe attack of encephalitis. Mabs grieved over the loss, as she never had much opportunity to enjoy true sisterhood while as she was away at school nine months out of the year, then relocating to attend Gallaudet.

After eight happy years in South Dakota, Mabs and Roy moved to the Tennessee School for the Deaf, in Knoxville, in 1955. They decided to further their educational studies in Special Education at the University of Tennessee, which was near the school. They enrolled for the Master's program during their first week of teaching at the school for the Deaf. During those years, their first son, Sam Kay, and their second son, Thomas Kay, were born in 1956 and 1959 in Knoxville, Tennessee. Mabs' parents moved to Knoxville to be near their grandsons. They looked after them while Mabs and Roy were at work and attending their graduate classes. Later Mabs and Roy were one of the first married couples to earn a second masters degree from California State University at Northridge under the National Leadership Training Program in 1968.

After that, Mabs finally broke out of the institutional teaching mold by going into teaching in a California public school in Santa Ana. Soon she was involved in post-secondary school instruction of the Deaf at Golden West College, Huntington Beach, California. In 1974, Roy accepted a Superintendent position in Delaware, at Margaret Sterck School for the Hearing Impaired in Newark. Mabs followed Roy a year later. While living in Delaware, Mabs was offered a position as manager of the statewide Deaf-Blind Search Program.

In 1977, both moved to California for special positions in the area of Deafness. At that time, Mabs took a teaching position at Ohone College in Fremont, and she later accepted a position directing a federally supported Regional Interpreter Training Program serving California, Nevada, Arizona and Utah.

During that time, while in his position with the Fremont school, Roy took care of his sons, functioning as a great "Mr. Mom." At the same time, both he and Mabs were grappling with the issue of "Total Communication." It was in 1967 that Roy advocated a new categorical concept, settling the controversy issue of Deaf communication modes, which became the philosophy of Total Communication. At the Forty-eight Conferences of Executives of American Schools for the Deaf in New York in 1976, it was officially adopted to have the many modes of communication used in the Deaf community housed under the label of Total Communication. Thus, Roy became known as the "Father of Total Communication," which earned him recognition. He was awarded an honorary doctorate degree from Gallaudet University, both for his leadership during the Total

Communication movement, and the fact that he founded International Association of the Parents of the Deaf (now better known as American Society of Deaf Children, or ASDC).

Mabs had interesting experiences accompanying Roy to many places, including visits to the International Congress of the Deaf in Sweden, in 1972, and then to Japan, in 1975. Roy was received with a standing ovation at both conferences.

During the years prior to 1985, as the first Director of the Gallaudet Regional Center at Ohlone College, Mabs expanded the qualification measures, which today stand as a tribute to her special abilities. She was also instrumental in the collaboration for the book "Deaf Women: A Parade through the Decades," which she co-authored with Sharon Kay Wood. Published by DawnSignPress in 1988, the book is recognized for it's uniqueness, as being the first book in the United States and the world, to focus primarily on the historical achievements of Deaf women. Mabs was a natural choice to co-author this book, due to her past involvement with the National Association of the Deaf (NAD) project of creating and developing a Deaf Women's Section under the NAD.

Health problems forced Mabs into early retirement in 1985. During a Deaf senior citizens social where members were introduced to tap dancing, Mabs discovered that she could not rotate her left ankle. When she accompanied Roy to his health specialist (Roy had Parkinson' s Disease), Mabs asked the doctor about her problem with rotating the ankle. The physician immediately had her examined and processed for brain surgery, as a tumor had been located that was pressing on her nervous system, causing partial paralysis of the left side of her body. Shortly after this discovery, during the

World Games of the Deaf in Los Angeles, many people stopped by to see the couple. They were shocked to see the impact the medical condition had on her. Mabs was baldheaded and partially paralyzed.

Despite her surgery and disability, it did not stop Mabs from writing more books, including *The Holcomb Heritage*, *The Pike Clan*, *The Brewster-Stakley Lineage*, and her autobiography, *The Sounds of Silence*.

Looking back on her life and her fifty years of companionship with Roy, who passed away in 1998, Mabs states that the years have been both great and challenging.

Mabs' story truly emphasizes the upbringing she received from a solid Deaf culture that has gone through many exciting and interesting changes. Such an experience has rarely been available to Deaf individuals. Mabs' life characterizes the early pioneering spirit of a highly qualified Deaf person shining brilliantly through a world dominated by hearing people.

Sharon Kay Wood was born in Lewinston, Idaho, and graduated from the Arizona School for the Deaf. She graduated from Gallaudet University with a BA in 1968, and obtained an MA in Deaf Education from New York University in 1983. Wood and Marjoriebell Holcomb co-authored the book, *Deaf Women: A Parade through the Decades*, published in 1989. Wood has been a teacher in schools for the Deaf for over 25 years. She currently lives in New Mexico with her husband, Henning Irgens, and is working on a second book about Deaf Women in the USA.

Henning C.F. Irgens was born in Oslo, Norway, and graduated from the Norwegian School for the Deaf. He earned a degree in Education, History and English from Gallaudet in 1957. Irgens, now retired, served the Michigan Department of Education as a Deaf Consultant. He also served as Project Director of Deaf Services at State Technical Institute in Michigan for more than 20 years. Currently, he serves as a member of the Board of Regents of the New Mexico School for the Deaf.

The husband and wife team often writes for various publications, and present at national and international conferences. Together, they adopted four dogs and two cats, most of them imported from Norway.

Sports Enthusiast

Anonymous

My mother is sixty-eight years old and a sports enthusiast. She attributes this characteristic to her school — the Trenton School for the Deaf. She often says,

"Trenton School, School for Deaf active, many do-do... softball, volleyball, basketball, and field hockey. Not like hearing school, people sit, sit all day talk, talk."

My mother played all these sports while in school, and also took up water skiing, downhill skiing, and tennis at about forty years of age. At fifty, she mastered slalom water skiing and continues to enjoy downhill skiing as well.

However, it's her tennis game that she is the most passionate about. She tried to teach me how to play tennis when I was in my twenties, but if there is ever a deterrent to playing tennis, it's having your mother teach you. That was the beginning and end of my tennis career. As noble as my mother's efforts to teach me how to be an athlete were, I took very little interest in playing, watching, or hearing about tennis. I didn't need a therapist to tell me that it was a combination of my mother's audible directions, and her somewhat demanding nature that ended my tennis career.

As a matter of fact, it wasn't only tennis that I avoided, it was the whole family altogether. After college, I moved 250 miles away to Boston and stayed there for five years. I moved back to New Jersey in my late twenties, and have remained there ever since. It shouldn't come as a surprise to any enlightened individual that while in Boston, I got a Master's Degree in Deaf Education. I have taught Deaf kids for ten years in Massachusetts, Pennsylvania, and New Jersey. So much for distancing myself from my family of origin!

Throughout the years, I have felt a wide range of emotion towards my mother, but I never did regard her as an "inspiration." I reserved that feeling for hearing women that I knew or read about who overcame prior hardships to achieve a level of personal or professional satisfaction and success.

A shift in my view began when my mother decided to sign up for a tennis tournament. Now, this was no ordinary tournament made up of regional Deaf clubs. My mother signed up for a tennis tournament featuring just about everyone in her hometown. At the age of sixty-five, she decided to compete against hearing women for the Senior Trophy. I couldn't believe it! My mother was going to compete against hearing people!

On top of all that, my mother set this up on her own and didn't ask me to interpret. I wasn't able to attend the matches, but received the results via TTY. According to my mother, her first opponent was fifty-five years old. As she described her opponent, "she short and fat, but strong." My mother lost the first set and was tied for the second when her opponent "FF'ed."

"What the heck that spell?" my mother asked.

"F-o-r-f-e-i-t mother, f-o-r-f-e-i-t," I replied.

And thus, my mother advanced to the second round, which was also the final round due to a shortage of players in her age bracket. She beat her second opponent with a solid 6-0, 6-1 victory. Imagine that! My mother was the reigning Senior Champion of her town. I realized it didn't matter that there were only a few opponents. The important thing was that my mother had achieved her goal: she had kicked some hearing butt.

At that moment, I found myself saying that my mother was an inspiration. And then it struck me like a bolt of lightning! The qualities leading to my mother's accomplishment — her courage, tenacity, and perseverance — were not recently developed. These qualities had been there all along. It just took me forty years to see them. Forty years to see that my mother is truly an inspiration.

About the Editors

Damara Goff Paris

Damara Goff Paris grew up in San Pablo, California, near the Bay Area. She lost her hearing at age two due to a vehicle accident. She moved to Oregon, where she graduated from Western Oregon University in 1994 with an MS in Rehabilitation Counseling in Deafness. While at Western, Damara received the "Most Distinguished Leadership Award" for her work in promoting campus access. She also received the "Best and Brightest Disabled College Graduate Award" from Mainstream Magazine, an award given to 10 individuals across the U.S.A. She obtained her NCC from the National Board of Certified Counselors in 1995.

Paris is currently the program manager of three state telecommunication assistance programs under Oregon Public Utility Commission. In addition to her duties for the state, Damara owns AGO Gifts and Publications. One of her publication projects focuses on Deaf Women in the Pacific Northwest. She is also a freelance writer for several other publications, including DeafNation Newspaper. Paris' community involvement includes serving as a board officer of the national Deaf Women United, Inc. and on the board of the Deaf and Hard of Hearing Access Program Advisory Board (DHHAP) in Salem, Oregon.

Paris is currently married to Joseph Paris and has one daughter, Sekoia Dawn Paris, born in April, 1998.

Mark Drolsbaugh

Mark Drolsbaugh is a graduate of Gallaudet graduate (BA in Psychology '92 and MA in School Counseling and Guidance, '94). After finishing his studies at Gallaudet, Drolsbaugh became a school counselor at the Pennsylvania School for the Deaf. In 1998, he won the Richard M. Phillips award for outstanding work by a Gallaudet alumnus in the Deaf community.

In addition to his school counselor duties, Drolsbaugh works at PSD's Center for Community and Professional Services (CCPS) as an AIDS Educator. Collaborating with a team of highly motivated professionals, Drolsbaugh works in the Philadelphia community advocating on behalf of AIDS awareness.

Shortly after joining PSD, Drolsbaugh began writing about his experiences as a Deaf individual. Eventually, he started a monthly column at DeafNation Newspaper.

Drolsbaugh published his first book, *Deaf Again*, in 1997. Deaf Again details his unusual experience of being born into a Deaf family, raised in the hearing world, and eventually rediscovering his Deaf identity upon attending Gallaudet University. The book has been recommended reading for a number of Deaf Culture/ASL classes throughout the United States, and has also done well overseas.

Drolsbaugh currently lives in Pennsylvania with his wife, Melanie, and his infant son, Darrin.

About the Illustrator
Wendell E. Goff

Wendell E. Goff was born in the San Francisco Bay area, and moved to Oregon with his family at the age of eight. At about three years of age, he contracted a viral fever, similar to Scarlet Fever, and sustained a substantial amount of hearing loss. Although he was severely hearing impaired, he became involved with music, collaborating with his father in the writing of country and gospel songs, and submitting them to publishing companies.

When he completely lost his hearing at twenty-three he turned to art as a means of expressing himself. He also learned sign language. He enrolled at Chemeteka Community College in the Visual Communications program. After one year there, he left for another year to work as a freelance news photographer before returning to school at Art Institutes International at Portland, Oregon. He is currently enrolled in the Computer Animation program and also accepts part-time graphic design work. He spends his free time with his four year old son, Conner Levi, as well as biking and dancing.

Two New Books from AGO Gifts and Publications!

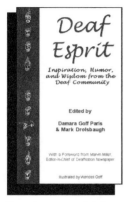

Imagine being Deaf and living through the German Occupation of Norway during World War II.

Learn about life among the Deaf Navajos.

Find out how a Deaf boy creates an ASL version of rock-scissors-paper.

Agonize with a mother as she tries to make sense of both sides of the cochlear implant controversy.

Laugh in the library with the well-known comedian, CJ Jones.

Penned by seasoned and new writers alike, with the goal of sharing the unique diversity in the Deaf community, *Deaf Esprit: Inspiration, Humor and Wisdom from the Deaf Community* edited by Damara Goff Paris and Mark Drolsbaugh, is a compilation of stories that will provoke a smile, a tear and, most important, a sense of well-being. Aptly named after the expression *"esprit de corps," Deaf Esprit* brings about the power of the spirit of the Deaf Community.

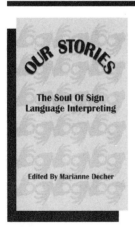

See our order form on the next page

Sign language interpreting is both an art and a science, with interpreters finding themselves uniquely between two worlds; a Deaf world in which most of them did not grow up as "natives", and a hearing world which has often not encountered interpreters and is unfamiliar with the profession. Aside from the myriad of personal histories and skills that interpreters, collectively, bring to their work, they are, above all, people working with people.

Our Stories: The Soul of Sign Language Interpreting edited by Marianne Decher, is the first book of its kind to look, not at the technical aspects of the field but rather, at the human side, at the people behind the profession.

From the light-hearted and humorous, to words of wisdom from a Deaf consumer, to an assignment that literally involved a life and death situation, various authors share their personal stories of what makes interpreting both challenging and rewarding.

AGO Gifts and Publications
ORDER FORM

Name: _____

Address: _____

City: _____

State: _____ Zip: _____

Payment Method:

____Check/Money Order ____Visa ____Mastercard

Card Number: _____

Expiration Date: _____

Signature (required):_____

Date of Order: _____

Order Information:
_____ "Our Stories" at $12.95 each for a total of: _____
_____ "Deaf Esprit" at $14.95 each for a total of: _____

Shipping and Handling: _____

TOTAL: _____

Shipping and Handling Rates:
1–5 books: $4.95   6–10 books: $6.95
11–20 books: $9.95   21–50 books: $12.95
*Over 50 books, contact for rates

Mail all orders to: **AGO Gifts and Publications**
                        P.O. Box 17664
                        Salem, Oregon 97305

Credit Card Orders may be faxed to: (503) 304-1961

Allow 4-6 weeks for delivery